# Psychiatric Mental Health Issues Within Healthcare

*Editor*

RENE LOVE

# NURSING CLINICS
# OF NORTH AMERICA

www.nursing.theclinics.com

*Consulting Editor*
STEPHEN D. KRAU

December 2019 • Volume 54 • Number 4

**ELSEVIER**

1600 John F. Kennedy Boulevard • Suite 1800 • Philadelphia, Pennsylvania, 19103-2899

http://www.theclinics.com

**NURSING CLINICS OF NORTH AMERICA Volume 54, Number 4**
**December 2019 ISSN 0029-6465, ISBN-13: 978-0-323-69658-6**

Editor: Kerry Holland
Developmental Editor: Nicole Congleton

*Nursing Clinics of North America* (ISSN 0029-6465) is published quarterly by Elsevier Inc., 360 Park Avenue South, New York, NY 10010-1710. Months of issue are March, June, September, and December. Periodicals postage paid at New York, NY and additional mailing offices. Subscription price per year is, $163.00 (US individuals), $491.00 (US institutions), $275.00 (international individuals), $598.00 (international institutions), $231.00 (Canadian individuals), $598.00 (Canadian institutions), $100.00 (US students), and $135.00 (international students). To receive student/resident rate, orders must be accompanied by name of affiliated institution, date of term, and the signature of program/residency coordinator on institution letterhead. Orders will be billed at individual rate until proof of status is received. Foreign air speed delivery is included in all *Clinics* subscription prices. All prices are subject to change without notice. **POSTMASTER:** Send address changes to *Nursing Clinics*, Elsevier Health Sciences Division, Subscription Customer Service, 3251 Riverport Lane, Maryland Heights, MO 63043. **Customer Service: Telephone: 1-800-654-2452** (U.S. and Canada); **1-314-447-8871 (outside U.S. and Canada). Fax: 1-314-447-8029. E-mail: journalscustomerservice-usa@elsevier.com** (for print support) and **journalsonlinesupport-usa@elsevier.com** (for online support).

*Nursing Clinics of North America* is covered in *EMBASE/Excerpta Medica, MEDLINE/PubMed (Index Medicus), Social Sciences Citation Index, Current Contents, ASCA, Cumulative Index to Nursing, RNdex Top 100,* and Allied Health Literature and International Nursing Index (INI).

# Contributors

## CONSULTING EDITOR

**STEPHEN D. KRAU, PhD, RN, CNE**
Associate Professor (Ret), Vanderbilt University School of Nursing, Nashville, Tennessee

## EDITOR

**RENE LOVE, PhD, DNP, PMHNP-BC, FNAP, FAANP**
DNP Director/Clinical Professor, The University of Arizona, College of Nursing, Tucson, Arizona

## AUTHORS

**BRITTANY ABELN, BSN, RN**
The University of Arizona, College of Nursing, Tucson, Arizona

**ELIZABETH BONHAM, PhD, RN, PMHCNS-BC, FAAN**
Associate Professor of Nursing, College of Nursing and Health Professions, University of Southern Indiana, Evansville, Indiana

**LINDSAY BOUCHARD, DNP, PMHNP-BC, RN**
Clinical Assistant Professor, College of Nursing, The University of Arizona, Tucson, Arizona

**CONNIE J. BRAYBROOK, DNP, PMHNP-BC**
United States Navy, Naval Branch Health Clinic Fallon, Fallon, Nevada

**JANE M. CARRINGTON, PhD, RN, FAAN**
Associate Professor, The University of Arizona, College of Nursing, Tucson, Arizona

**JADE MONTANEZ CHATMAN, BSN, RN**
PhD Student, Doctoral Student, School of Nursing, University of Louisville, Louisville, Kentucky

**DANA W. CONVOY, BSN, RN-C**
Commander, United States Navy Reserve, Naval Operation Support Center, Wilmington, North Carolina

**SEAN P. CONVOY, DNP, PMHNP-BC**
Assistant Professor, Duke University School of Nursing, Durham, North Carolina

**CHRISTINE B. COSTA, DNP, PMHNP-BC**
Assistant Professor, School of Nursing, California State University Long Beach, Long Beach, California

**CATHLEEN M. DECKERS, EdD, RN**
Assistant Professor, California State University, Long Beach, School of Nursing, Long Beach, California

**SATTARIA DILKS, DNP, PMHNP-BC**
Professor, McNeese State University, College of Nursing and Health Professions, Lake Charles, Louisiana

**GAYLE J. EARLY, PhD, FNP-BC**
Assistant Professor, California State University, Long Beach, School of Nursing, Long Beach, California

**SOPHIA D. FALANA, BSN, RN**
DNP-PMHNP Student, The University of Arizona, College of Nursing, Tucson, Arizona

**LINDA SUE HAMMONDS, DNP, PMHNP-BC, FNP**
Department of Community Mental Health, University of South Alabama, Assistant Professor, College of Nursing, Mobile, Alabama

**CARLA HERMANN, PhD, RN**
Professor, MSN Program Director, Indiana University Southeast, School of Nursing, New Albany, Indiana

**VICKI HINES-MARTIN, PhD, PMHCNS, RN, FAAN**
Professor, School of Nursing, University of Louisville, Louisville, Kentucky

**JESSICA JOHNSON, PhD, MSN**
Neurocrine Bioscience, Inc., San Diego, California

**CRYSTAL KELLY, MSN, FNP**
Neurocrine Bioscience, Inc., San Diego, California

**ASHLEY S. LOVE, DNP, PMHNP-BC**
Serenity Psychiatric Care, Benson Health Clinic, Eugene, Oregon

**RENE LOVE, PhD, DNP, PMHNP-BC, FNAP, FAANP**
DNP Director/Clinical Professor, The University of Arizona, College of Nursing, Tucson, Arizona

**KATHLEEN T. McCOY, DNSc, APRN, PMHNP-BC, PMHCNS-BC, FNP-BC, FAANP**
Associate Professor, Department of Community Mental Health, University of South Alabama, College of Nursing, Mobile, Alabama

**KIRSTEN PANCIONE, DNP, PMHNP-BC, FNP-BC**
Department of Community Mental Health, University of South Alabama, Assistant Professor, College of Nursing, Mobile, Alabama

**EVELYN PARRISH, PhD, PMHNP-BC, FAANP**
Associate Professor and Director of Accreditation and Strategic Outcomes, University of Kentucky College of Nursing, Lexington, Kentucky

**MONTRAY SMITH, MSN, MPH, RN, LHRM**
Doctoral Student, School of Nursing, University of Louisville, Louisville, Kentucky

**SHAQUITA STARKS, PhD, RN, APRN, FNP-BC, PMHNP-BC**
Assistant Professor, Department of Health Promotion and Disease Prevention, Advanced Practice and Doctoral Studies, College of Nursing, The University of Tennessee, The University of Tennessee Health Sciences Center, Memphis, Tennessee

**IAN THOMAS, DNP, PMHNP**
Psychiatric Nurse Practitioner, Carondelet Health Network, Tucson, Arizona

**PAMELA HERBIG WALL, PhD, PMHNP-BC, FAANP**
Consulting Associate, United States Government, Sanford, North Carolina

**RICHARD J. WESTPHAL, PhD, PMHNP-BC, PMHCNS-BC, FAAN**
Professor of Nursing, Woodward Clinical Scholar, University of Virginia at Charlottesville, Charlottesville, Virginia

**ROSE MARY XAVIER, PhD, MS, PMHNP-BC**
Assistant Professor, The University of North Carolina at Chapel Hill, School of Nursing, Chapel Hill, North Carolina

# Contents

veteran populations. This article explores the pathophysiology, identification, and treatment of military service–connected trauma-related and stressor-related disorders. Particular attention is given to trauma informed care, evidence-based practice recommendations, and the sequencing of psychotherapy and pharmacotherapy in pursuit of optimal patient outcomes.

Management of attention-deficit/hyperactivity disorders require provider skill, rapport, and referral acumen to treat patients across the life span. Incidence and prevalence have increased in the United States and globally. There are innovative models of evidence-informed screening techniques, treatment strategies to help providers work with patients and their families. Diplomatic management of highly charged treatment controversies, drug diversion, and risk factor reduction helps to ethically address this growing public health phenomenon. This article examines risk factors and treatment considerations in the United States for evidence-informed care, with a focus on affordable and readily accessible treatment in primary care settings.

This article offers an alternative conceptualization from which a health care provider can consider and respond to client-based suicidal ideation and behavior. Pragmatically explored through the prism of locus of control, Rogerian psychotherapy principles, Peplau's theory of interpersonal relations, and the work of Kay Redfield Jamison, the Concordant Actions in Suicide Assessment (CASA) model frames clinical decision making along a continuum defined by concordant and state-based action. Therein, cognitive reframes are offered to illustrate how to apply the CASA model in clinical practice.

Delirium superimposed on dementia is an acute medical illness that is difficult to diagnose because of the similarities of the symptoms to dementia. Delirium can contribute to the suffering of the patient as well as the family and caregiver. An initial holistic assessment of the patient is critical in establishing the cognitive baseline symptoms of delirium. Prevention of delirium can be assisted by ongoing reassessment of the patient for symptoms of delirium. The goal of treatment is to treat the underlying cause of the delirium.

Transgender individuals are at an increased risk of experiencing health inequalities, such as anxiety, depression, and HIV. It is important that providers and staff in the health care setting are prepared to care for this population to ensure best patient outcomes. An understanding of transgender terminology and the experience of gender dysphoria is key. In addition, a transinclusive environment should be created to reduce the likelihood of transgender-related discrimination. Developing an understanding of potential gender-affirming treatments and surgeries also optimizes patient care. Improving the quality care will reduce health disparities commonly faced by the transgender population.

Postpartum depression (PPD) affects10% to 20% of women within the first year after birth and 25% beyond the first year. PPD, despite advances in diagnosis and treatment, remains underdiagnosed and misunderstood. Women do not always display signs of PPD while in care for delivery of the infant and may not discuss mood changes to their primary care provider at discharge and first post-delivery appointment. Identifying screening and treatment options for non–mental health providers was the purpose of this article.

Human trafficking is the intentional exploitation of vulnerable individuals for the personal gain of the exploiter and is now recognized as an emerging public health care priority. Health care providers are well positioned to identify and assist trafficked individuals as well as those who may be at risk for exploitation. Trauma informed care is essential to identify victims and evaluate the impact of traumatic stress while highlighting survivors' strengths and supporting their resiliency. Human trafficking demographics, including mental and physical health problems, health considerations, risk factors, screening, implications for practice, and national resources, are reviewed.

The trajectory of human development follows a predictable course of milestones. As genomic research has brought us more understanding of the brain, the etiology of mental illness is progressing from psychodynamic origins postulated by Freud in 1960 to organic pathways and epigenetic derivations. Humans develop on normal pathways that can be derailed by poverty, illness, and trauma. When infants begin life from a healthy perspective, conditions that may follow such as a mental disorder may be moderated by healthy starts. In this paper, selected developmental theories and mental disorders are presented; then their interface is discussed. Implications for nursing are outlined.

Antipsychotics can be life changing, but like all medications, they can also have unwanted effects, including drug-induced movement disorders such as tardive dyskinesia (TD). More patients are receiving antipsychotic treatment from non-psychiatry health care providers, including primary care and general practitioners. Despite misconceptions to the contrary, recent analyses suggest that the risk of drug-induced movement disorders such as TD has not been eliminated. Nurses across all care settings will increasingly encounter patients treated with antipsychotics. Nurses are critical for ensuring that patients exposed to antipsychotics receive screening and monitoring, care, and education.

The impact of culture on health has gained considerable importance in care delivery. This review discusses the complex interaction of culture and social determinants, and the combined impact of these on emotional well-being. Examples of this interaction are presented and recommendations for change within nursing to improve care are discussed.

Compassion fatigue (CF) can be detrimental to health care providers' mental and physical health, efficiency, and quality of patient care. Although many studies explore CF in physicians and nurses, there is currently limited published research regarding how advanced practice registered nurses (APRNs) develop and address CF. APRNs may be at high risk for developing CF due to their work responsibilities, patient interaction, and personal characteristics. Because of its impact on health care providers, patients, and organizations, APRNs should be aware of the potential causes, symptoms, and negative effects of this phenomenon.

# NURSING CLINICS OF NORTH AMERICA

**SERIES OF RELATED INTEREST**

*Critical Care Nursing*
Available at: https://www.ccnursing.theclinics.com/

**THE CLINICS ARE AVAILABLE ONLINE!**
Access your subscription at:
www.theclinics.com

# NURSING CLINICS OF
# NORTH AMERICA

FORTHCOMING ISSUES

March 2026
Leading Innovative Nurse-Leaders in the
Point of Care
Kelly A. Wolgast, Editor

June 2026
Workplace Bullying
Renee Thompson, Editor

September 2026
Cancer Prevention and Detection
Pamela S. Hinds, Editor

RECENT ISSUES

September 2025
Transitions of Care in Pediatric Nursing
Anna Goddard, Editor
Gregory S. Knudson, Editor

June 2025
Infectious Diseases
Randolph F.R. Rasch, Editor

March 2025

# Foreword

# Psychiatric Disorders

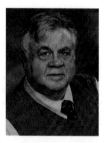

Stephen D. Krau, PhD, RN, CNE
*Consulting Editor*

Mental Health emerges to the forefront of everyone's mind when certain violent atrocities occur. In a feeble effort to logically explain horrible behaviors, mental health becomes a topic and is called to reconcile the illogical and perverse behaviors to logic. This holds not only for the violent outrages but also for many social struggles for which there is no easy comprehension. Among those readily encountered include but are not limited to the "opioid epidemic," homeless persons, and the myriad of violent behaviors readily conveyed in all forms of media. It is clear mental health and mental health issues either directly or indirectly affect us all. This affects us not only as nurses, medical professionals, and caretakers, but equally as citizens of global inhabitants. As this is the case, it begs the question as to why mental health does not get the attention it deserves until there is an emergent crisis, issue, or social problem.

Mental disorders have been studied, and findings indicate that reported global prevalence is between 12.2% and 48.6%.[1] Tomlinson and Lund[2] have reviewed the problem and confirm that mental health focus, despite the global burden, is not commensurate to its visibility, policy attention, or funding. They apply a framework proposed by Shiffman and Smith[2,3] for an analysis to explain why some global health initiatives are more successful in generating funding and political focus than others. Although predominately applied to maternal child health nursing, the framework is instrumental in examining priorities in mental health funding and political prioritization of mental health. Their focus has been global health, and it has been successful. The point here is not to adulterate their superb model, but rather to present the model such that its tenets and principles are applicable to mental health issues at the national, state, and local levels. The extent to which health care professionals, as opposed to politicians, are engaged at these levels, remains uncertain. There are, nonetheless, opportunities for nurses and other health care professionals to be involved.

Shiffman and Smith[3] have identified that when 3 conditions are met, that the health issue becomes a political priority. One condition that is essential is the attention to the

https://doi.org/10.1016/j.cnur.2019.09.001
0029-6465/19/© 2019 Published by Elsevier Inc.

**Table 1**
**Four components of Shiffman and Smith's framework**

| Actor Power | Description of the Issue | Context of Actors' Actions | Characteristics of the Issue Itself |
|---|---|---|---|
| Cohesive leadership | How issue is characterized | Environment in which actors operate | Extent to which credible indicators exist |
| Guiding institution or body | How issue is described | Ability of actors to take advantage of windows | Indicators to assess and monitor progress |
| Mobilization of civil society | These work to draw attention to the issue | Goal to influence decision makers | Evidence interventions are cost-effective and can be implemented at scale |

*Data from* Shiffman J, Smith S. Generation of political priority for global health initiatives: a framework and case study of maternal mortality. Lancet 2007;370(9595):1370-9.

issue from political leaders as well as international leaders in support of the issue in a manner that is ongoing and *sustained*. It is essential that support does not just emerge in the presence of a crisis, or the emergence of a violent atrocity. In addition, it is imperative that there are existing and enacted policies that address the issue, in this case mental health. Equally important is that resources are allocated to the issue appropriately to the disease burden. None of these conditions are being met globally in a substantial manner when it comes to mental health.[2] At the national level, it waivers, as state and local levels show no consistency or norm.

The Shiffman and Smith framework also includes 4 components as presented in **Table 1**.

The utilization of this model is apparent with regard to disease processes that are clear, with internationally accepted measurements and standards. In addition, the framework is more utilized in processes deemed more urgent when lives are immediately at stake, such as newborn diseases, AIDS, and such. With mental health issues, there needs to be a stronger voice, and more agreement on empirical indicators and measurements of mental health diseases. It would seem that part of the issue is the disparity in measurement versus opinions in the field of mental health. In addition, the stigma associated with mental health is a deterrent to discussing, exploring, and dealing with these issues.[1]

Other factors impacting the advancement of mental health interventions include questionable social justice and human rights framework. The extent to which health is perceived as a human right is the fodder of much debate. It is hoped that health care providers will be included among the "actors" in this model so that we can move forward in a permanent and consistent manner for the benefit of us all.

Stephen D. Krau, PhD, RN, CNE
Vanderbilt University School of Nursing
6809 Highland Park Drive
Nashville, TN 37205, USA

*E-mail address:*
sbluefountain@aol.com

## REFERENCES

1. World Health Organization. Cross-national comparisons of the prevalences and correlates of mental disorders. WHO International Consortium in Psychiatric Epidemiology. Bull World Health Organ 2000;78:413–26.
2. Tomlinson M, Lund C. Why does mental health not get the attention it deserves? An application of the Shiffman and Smith framework. PLoS Med 2012;9(2):e1001178. Available at: https://doi.org/10.1371/journal.pmed.1001178. Accessed September 1, 2019.
3. Shiffman J, Smith S. Generation of political priority for global health initiatives: a framework and case study of maternal mortality. Lancet 2007;370:1370–9. Available at: https://papers.ssrn.com/sol3/papers.cfm?abstract_id=1101659. Accessed September 1, 2019.

# Preface

# Psychiatric Mental Health Issues Within Primary and Acute Care Settings

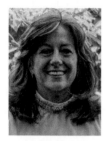

Rene Love, PhD, DNP, PMHNP-BC, FNAP, FAANP
*Editor*

As the landscape in health care is changing, more patients are being seen by their primary care providers and in hospitals for psychiatric mental health disorders. This is due in part to an increase in demand for psychiatric mental health services. As stigma decreases around mental health disorders in combination with the lack of access to Psychiatric Mental Health providers, primary care and acute care providers are addressing these disorders in their practice setting. In addition, patients may also be more comfortable talking with their established providers about their mental health concerns. While addressing these concerns is helpful, it puts an additional burden on nonmental health providers.

Based on these concerns, this special issue addresses multiple topics on psychiatric disorders and concerns that may occur in your practice setting. Topics such as anxiety, depression, posttraumatic stress disorder, Attention-deficit/hyperactivity disorder, postpartum depression, suicidal patients, and substance abuse are addressed in this special issue. This special issue will also address other topics encountered, such as human trafficking, developmental behavioral issues, compassion fatigue, and cultural diversity. We also looked at topics, such as prescribing antipsychotic medication and how to tell the difference between dementia and delirium. It is hoped that these topics will answer some of the questions that have arisen for you while working in your practice setting.

The best of all care aligns when providers work in collaboration or consultation to provide the most effective and efficient outcomes for the patient. Interprofessional practices are becoming more and more common with shared electronic health records and team meetings. This type of practice setting allows for consultations and warm handoffs of troubled patients, allowing the providers to view and understand the

Nurs Clin N Am 54 (2019) xvii–xviii
https://doi.org/10.1016/j.cnur.2019.08.009
0029-6465/19/© 2019 Published by Elsevier Inc.

patient's issues from both the physical and the mental health perspective. It is hoped that this type of practice setting will continue to grow to support providers while improving care to the patient.

It is my hope that this special issue of *Nursing Clinics of North America* will improve patient care as well as provide foundational knowledge for providers. Like all aspects of care for patients, the specialty of psychiatric mental health is evolving at a fast speed as evidenced by the Food and Drug Administration's approval for a medication for postpartum depression since the development of the articles. The improved treatment options for mental health disorders is very exciting and requires us to continually stay updated using evidence-based practice knowledge with all patients.

Rene Love, PhD, DNP, PMHNP-BC, FNAP, FAANP
University of Arizona
1305 North Martin Avenue
Tucson, AZ 85721, USA

*E-mail address:*
renelove@email.arizona.edu

# Anticipating Changes for Depression Management in Primary Care

Kathleen T. McCoy, DNSc, APRN, PMHNP-BC, PMHCNS-BC, FNP-BC, FAANP[a],*,
Christine B. Costa, DNP, PMHNP-BC[b],
Kirsten Pancione, DNP, PMHNP-BC, FNP-BC[a,1],
Linda Sue Hammonds, DNP, PMHNP-BC, FNP[a,2]

## KEYWORDS

- Depression • Telehealth • Wellness-based reimbursement initiative
- Measurement based care • Pharmacogenetics • Integrative care model

## KEY POINTS

- Depressive clinical presentations are diverse, including lack of sad affect for various reasons, and normative for culture presentation(s).
- Measurement-based care as standard for usual practice is an emerging practice.
- There is increased drive for wellness care versus encounter-based care.
- Telehealth offers the unique ability to increase access to care.
- The integrative care model shows promising potential to avoid treatment disruption and ensure continuity of care.

## INTRODUCTION

Depression is a global issue, according to the World Health Organization (WHO), exceeding 300 million people affected, an increase of 18% between 2005 and 2015.[1] As reported by Pratt and Brody in 2014,[2] US households have some 7.6% depressed persons aged 12 years and over, with moderate or severe depressive symptoms, with women more often affected than men. In that report, those living below the poverty line have increased occurrence of depression. With only 35% of those seeking treatment with mental health professionals within the last year, leaving

Disclosure: The authors have nothing to disclose.
[a] Department of Community Mental Health, University of South Alabama, HAHN 3044, 5721 USA Drive North, Mobile, AL 36688-0002, USA; [b] College of Nursing, California State University, Long Beach, 1250 Bellflower Boulevard MS 0301, Long Beach, CA 90804, USA
[1] Present address: 13707 Ishnala Circle, Wellington, FL 33414.
[2] Present address: 287 Sunny Valley Lane, Poplar Bluff, MO 63901.
* Corresponding author. 534 Ridgecrest Drive, McMinnville, TN 37110.
E-mail address: mccoy@southalabama.edu

Nurs Clin N Am 54 (2019) 457–471
https://doi.org/10.1016/j.cnur.2019.07.001
0029-6465/19/© 2019 Elsevier Inc. All rights reserved.
nursing.theclinics.com

the remainder as untreated, or treated in primary care. Because depression has affective, cognitive, and somatic effects, it is important for providers to be able to diagnose, treat and/or refer in a timely manner for good clinical outcomes.[2] Halverson and colleagues[3] reported that most patients with depression present initially in primary care settings. Common clinical presentations, appropriate treatment, and the changing dynamics for the care of patients with depression in primary care settings are reviewed in this article.

## CAUSES OF DEPRESSION

There are different biological and psychosocial theories related to the causes of depression. The course of the illness varies significantly with age of onset, biological factors, environmental and personal vulnerabilities, such as poverty, loss, or series of losses (spousal, death of loved one/significant other), or sudden physiologic/psychological insult, such as motor vehicle accident(s) and financial issues.[4] Comorbid mental and medical disorders, including those of idiopathic origin, exacerbate the clinical course of illness.

## INCIDENCE

The incidence of depression in the global population, as reported by WHO in 2015, was estimated to be 4.4%.[1] Depression is more often found in women (5.1%) than in men (3.6%). Its prevalence varies from a low 2.6% among men in the Western Pacific Region to 5.9% among women in the African Region. Prevalence rates vary by age, peaking in older adulthood (above 7.5% among women, and above 5.5% among men, aged 55–74 years). Childhood depression in those under the age of 15 years is more common than in those over the age of 15 years. Globally, 322 million people suffer with depression, with almost half of these individuals residing in the South-East Asia Region and the Western Pacific Region, including India and China. This increase of 18.4% from 2005 to 2015, reflects the overall global population increase. Globally, depressive disorders are ranked as the single largest contributor to non-fatal health loss, and contribute to 7.5% of all *Years Lost to Disability* reports. Suicide is more prevalent in lower-income nations than in middle- to high-income nations, is seen in men more than in women, and peaks between the ages of 17 and 20 years, and gradually levels off across the lifespan.

Brody and Pratt[2] reported that, between 2013 and 2016, of 8.1% of adults with depression in the US, in a given 2-week period, the incidence of women with depression was twice that in men. Age did not change prevalence, but culture had a bearing: non-Hispanic Asian adults had the lowest prevalence of depression, and this prevalence did not vary significantly among other races and Hispanic-origin groups studied. The low-income variable increases the occurrence of depression in proportion to the extent of experiences of poverty at the family income level. Approximately 80% of depressed adults report functional impairments (work, home, and social activities) because of symptoms. Depression rates by sex in the US, from 2007–2008 to 2015–2016, show no significant changes. Mojtabai and colleagues[5] investigated the prevalence of major depressive disorder among school-age children aged 12 to 17 years, noting a significant increase in the previous decade: 8.7% in 2005 to 11.5% in 2014, and a 37% surge in major depressive disorder among school-age children. In 2018, WHO reported, globally, an estimated 53,000 deaths by suicide in school-age children in 2016, making suicide the third leading cause of death in 15- to 19-year-olds; second leading cause of death in women in this age group.[6]

## PATHOPHYSIOLOGY

Science has moved from the pure monoamine theory of depression, as per Goldberg and colleagues[7] and McEwen's[8] publications in the Annals of the New York Academy of Science, to the theory of linked connections between elevated hypothalamic-pituitary-adrenal axis activity and protracted stress consideration. The complexity and heterogeneity of depression, as described by Duman,[9] defies a simple under-standing of the pathophysiology of depression, and through new and fast-acting novel treatments, some pathways are more easily seen. Among the stress/depression associations with neuronal atrophy, with its characteristic loss of limbic and cortical synaptic connections, it is thought that concomitant decreased expression of hippo-campal and prefrontal cortex brain-derived neurotrophic factor (BDNF) occurs. More recent studies have elucidated the role of glutamate and its transmission, followed by changes in BDNF, causing downstream signaling and reducing stimulation of synap-ses and concomitant reduction of brain functioning.

## THEORY

Alterations in synaptogenesis and neural plasticity cause functional disconnections, which underly the pathophysiology (and treatment) of depression.[9] The results are neuronal atrophy, resulting in problems in the signaling pathways caused by stress and depression. Neurotrophic factors, proinflammatory cytokines, sex steroids, meta-bolic/feeding factors (ie, insulin/diabetes, leptin, and ghrelin), among other factors, play a role in depression and its alleviation. With several causes merging, including the stress diathesis of McEwen,[8] it is clear that there is no one straight path to depres-sion, and depression may result from cumulative responses to multiple influences.

## SOCIAL DETERMINANTS OF MENTAL HEALTH

Social context influences the development and course of mental illness. According to WHO, social determinants of health, or conditions in which individuals "are born, grow, live, work and age," are influenced by economic status, social power, and access to resources such as education, health, and safe environments.[10] Determinants for mental health include discrimination, adverse early life experiences, lack of and/or poor education, unemployment, poverty, food insecurity, housing instability, adverse housing, and poor access to health care, and these cause cumulative physical and psy-chological stress over time, resulting in systematic differences in mental health develop-ment and prognosis. Such factors are part and parcel of case formulations for depressed patients to reduce impacts by acting on social determinants in care planning.

Awareness of intersecting effects of race, gender, and socioeconomic status on depression is important.[11] For example, whether income operates as a risk or protective factor for patients with depression depends on these and other socioeco-nomic characteristics. Because higher rates of depression are seen in lower-socioeconomic populations, predictions of higher risk for these populations, as well as adverse consequences and poor treatment outcomes, are outlined below. Frame-works created to incorporate social determinants of health provide a more complete picture of why people become ill initially, and what it takes to readily access quality health care, targeted to individual health outcomes.[12]

## INTERPLAY OF SOCIAL DETERMINANTS OF HEALTH ON DEPRESSION OUTCOMES

- White women benefit from higher income and the residual effect of high income (above and beyond education, employment, and marital status).

- Race (African American) and high household income has been found to be protective against risk of 12-month major depressive episode.
- Larger mental health gain from household income for women than men.
- High household income was protective for Caucasian women, and high education was protective for African American women.
- High income is a risk factor for depression in African American men after controlling for effects of other socioeconomic indicators.[12]

## PRIMARY CARE SCREENING FOR SOCIAL DETERMINANTS

Screening for social determinants of health helps identify patients who may benefit from greater support in one or more areas, thus promoting a holistic, public health approach, especially for those individuals who come from marginalized and underserved backgrounds. These factors are closely linked to health outcomes. The growing body of evidence supports social screening and intervention in primary care, while recognizing the need to continue developing and refining available screening tools and interventions. It is important to take more complete health histories, screening for social and environmental determinants of mental health in primary care, including identifying factors such as: family history of depression, adverse early life experiences, maternal stress during pregnancy, unemployment, food insecurity, poor education, and homelessness/housing instability, discrimination, and domestic/intimate partner violence. Screening for social determinants of health in clinical care includes health-related behaviors such as poor nutrition, excessive drinking, substance use, and physical inactivity.[12]

## POLICY CHANGE

Policy changes to alleviate social determinants of health, such as poverty, racism, violence, and lack of access to resources, can have far-reaching impacts in improving the health of a community, state, or nation. Although there are no universal screening requirements for social determinants, addressing only the symptoms of illness and ignoring root causation will not improve population health. Screening benefits include providing whole-person care and more accurate diagnosis. Understanding important information in terms of living conditions and social context, reduces recurrent emergency room visits by addressing the underlying causes of illness and decreases costs through early intervention, increasing adherence to treatment regimens, and providing more trauma-informed care. In operationalizing effective screening for social determinants of health in clinical care, good clinical outcomes move from the "margins to the mainstream."[13]

## GENERAL POPULATION PRESENTATION OF MAJOR DEPRESSIVE DISORDER

There are many variations and levels of depression (**Table 1**). Major depressive disorder is the generic depression discussed. Patients presenting with less than full criteria should still be considered for appropriate therapeutic management. Symptom presentation in children/adolescents varies slightly with increased irritability being a typical presentation seen by family, friends, and providers.[28] Other high-risk populations vulnerable to depression include those with substance abuse, the elderly, and postpartum women. Postpartum depression and/or psychosis are high risk for those with a previous history of depression, as are bipolar states because of disturbances in sleep cycle, changing family dynamics, and high biological flux.[10] Depression in the elderly can often be overlooked due to somatic presentations, the ageing process, and increasing frailty. In this age group,

**Table 1**
**Across the lifespan clinical presentation/evidence for depression with developmentally appropriate evidence informed screening instrument**

| Lifespan Population-Based Symptoms of Depression | Screening Instruments |
| --- | --- |
| General population<br>Symptoms must be present during the same 2-week period, representing a change in functioning to include either depressed mood and/or loss of interest or pleasure that are clearly not attributable to another disorder and 5 or more of the following per the American Psychological Association[14]<br>• Depressed mood most of the day, most days, either by subjective report (sad, empty, hopeless) or observable by others<br>• Marked diminished interest, pleasure, in all or almost all, activities most of the day, every day either by report of self/others<br>• Significant weight loss not related to dieting (5% change in body weight/month) or appetite decrease nearly daily or weight gain<br>• Insomnia or hypersomnia nearly daily<br>• Psychomotor agitation or retardation nearly every day<br>• Fatigue or loss of energy nearly every day<br>• Feelings of worthlessness or excessive guilt nearly daily<br>• Lowered ability to think, concentrate or indecisiveness, nearly daily<br>• Recurrent thoughts of death, recurrent suicidal ideation without a specific plan, or attempt or a specific plan for committing suicide | Mood Disorder Questionnaire (MDQ) for adults https://www.integration.samhsa.gov/clinical-practice/screening-tools[15]<br>PHQ-9 https://www.uspreventiveservicestaskforce.org/Home/GetFileByID/218[16]<br>PRIME-MD Patient Health Questionnaire (PHQ) http://www.oacbdd.org/clientuploads/Docs/2010/Spring%20Handouts/Session%20220j.pdf[17] |
| Hallmark school-age presentation of depression[15]<br>• Irritability<br>• Fatigue (somatic complaints)<br>• Insomnia or sleeping more<br>• Decline in academic functioning | Pediatric Symptom Checklist (PSC-17) https://www.brightfutures.org/mentalhealth/pdf/professionals/ped_sympton_chklst.pdf[18]<br>Columbia Suicide Severity Rating Scale (CSSRS) https://cssrs.columbia.edu/wp-content/uploads/C-SSRS_Pediatric-SLC_11.14.16.pdf[19] |
| Hallmark presentation of depression with substance use<br>• Symptoms of depression are not due to direct physiologic effects of substance<br>• Symptoms and history should be weighed carefully together in the diagnostic assessment<br>• Referral for treatment of substance use<br>• 2-wk duration depressed mood/loss of interest before use of substance or abstinence free of substance[16,17] | CAGE-AID http://www.integration.samhsa.gov/images/res/CAGEAID.pdf[20]<br>Beck Depression Inventory (BDI) https://www.apa.org/pi/about/publications/caregivers/pra ctice-settings/assessment/tools/beck-depression.aspx[21] |

(continued on next page)

| Table 1 (continued) | |
|---|---|
| **Lifespan Population-Based Symptoms of Depression** | **Screening Instruments** |
| Hallmark presentation of depression for women of childbearing age<br>• Non-gravid: see DSM-5 description (see **Box 1**) (excepting those with premenstrual-related disorders and other differential diagnosis)<br>• Gravid:<br>  ○ More emotional lability per Fischer (2018) than non-gravid counterparts<br>  ○ 50% of pregnancies in the United States are unplanned as per Bonham, The Shriver Report (2018)<br>  ○ 60% of pregnancies in the bipolar population are unplanned per Rusner et al<br>• Postpartum:<br>  ○ Spousal/family upheaval<br>  ○ Financial upheaval<br>  ○ General biological flux, hormonal, sleep, lactation, pain, weight issues<br>• Menopausal:<br>  ○ Mood changes common<br>  ○ If more than normal, seek solutions through the North American Menopause Society<br>  ○ Screen for depression<br>  ○ Antidepressants and psychotherapy/counseling combinations recommended (NAMS) | For women of childbearing age:<br>Massachusetts General Hospital https://womensmentalhealth.org/[22]<br>For all pregnant women wk 26 through 6 wk postpartum:<br>Edinburgh Postpartum Depression Scale (EPDS) https://www.knowppd.com/epds-ppd-screening/[23]<br>For peri-menopausal women:<br>https://www.menopause.org/for-women/menopauseflashes/mental-health-at-menopause/depression-menopause[24,25] |
| Hallmark elderly presentation of depression<br>• Depressive mood<br>• Loss of interest/desire<br>  ○ Anhedonia<br>• Excessive feelings of guilt<br>• Psychomotor<br>  ○ Agitation, retardation | Geriatric Depression Scale (GDS) https://consultgeri.org/try-this/general-assessment/issue-4.pdf[26] |
| • Vegetative symptoms<br>  Sleepiness, loss of appetite, insomnia<br>• Somatic symptoms<br>  Headaches, backaches, gastrointestinal, pain<br>• Cognitive symptoms<br>  Dullness, indecision | Geriatric Depression Scale-15 http://geriatrictoolkit.missouri.edu/cog/GDS_SHORT_FORM.PDF[27] |

Data from Refs.[14–24,26]

subthreshold symptoms can cause loss of functionality (see Fiske and colleagues).[28]

## CLINICAL TREATMENT GOALS: REMISSION OF SYMPTOMS

Depression is treatable, with many paths to recovery, as outlined in **Box 1**. Unfortunately, true remission is generally unsought, with "less than" recovery generally

| Box 1 |
| :-- |
| **Medication treatment implications/strategies** |

| Lifespan Presentations | Psychopharmacologic |
| :-- | :-- |
| Adult (general population) | Selective serotonin reuptake inhibitor (SSRIs), serotonin-norepinephrine reuptake inhibitor (SNRIs), buspirone, lithium, and thyroid as augmentation strategies, newer atypical antipsychotic formulations |
| School age | • Start low, go slow<br>• First line: fluoxetine plus therapy<br>• Second line: sertraline or lexapro<br>• Third line: venlafaxine<br>• May consider bupropion or duloxetine after venlafaxine<br>• Close monitoring essential secondary to risk of bipolar exacerbation vs suicide<br><br>Pharmacologic considerations are important in school age youth despite negative media coverage 2004–2006 and US Food and Drug Administration (FDA) initiation of black box warnings of all SSRIs of potential increased risk of suicide in youths, SSRI youth prescription rates dropped 20%, culminating in the largest increase in the Centers for Disease Control and Prevention (CDC) report on school-age suicides (2011), stressing the importance that evidence shows SSRIs are safe and effective if closely monitored. All adolescent post mortem toxicology reports are absent of antidepressants despite being prescribed.[29–31] |
| Substance use | • Certain SSRIs, SNRIs, buspirone, most likely patient has had previous trials, rule out bipolar mood disorder<br>• Considerations of comorbid attention-deficit/hyperactivity disorder and/or acute/chronic pain syndromes and pregnancy<br>• Awareness of prescription medication abuse: gabapentin, diphenhydramine, quetiapine, carisoprodol, clonidine, and ibuprofen[32] |
| Women of childbearing age | Providers must be updated/aware of the following contingencies (Massachusetts General Hospital):<br><br>• Collaboration with obstetrician and essential early prenatal care<br>• Birth control vs fertility consideration<br>• Planned vs unplanned pregnancy/and risks associated<br>• Consider psychotherapies plus low-risk medicines<br>• No alcohol secondary to fetal birth defects<br>• Risks vs benefits of pharmacologic treatment during pregnancy/postpartum time<br>• Folate as precaution<br>• Pregnancy/opioid issues: methadone/buprenorphine (sole)<br>• The new US FDA Pregnancy Labeling and Lactation Rule<br>• Screening: evidence-informed screening lends to more accurate diagnosis and treatment, saving time and resources to recovery<br>• Risk of neonatal symptoms, long-term effects, antidepressant risk, SSRI risks, persistent pulmonary hypertension of the newborn vs development of postpartum depression/psychosis[22] |
| Elderly | • Need for prescribing antidepressants for elderly to be evidence based<br>• Start low, go slow<br>• Avoid drug-drug interactions<br>• Early screening/intervention for delirium onset<br>• Screening Tool of Older People's Prescriptions (STOPP)[33]<br>• BEERS Criteria[34] |
| Genetic pharmacologic testing | Genetic pharmacologic testing as a time savings for treatment efficacy. This area is promising but limited. Rosenblat and colleagues[35] completed a meta-analysis finding evidence to be limited and with methodological deficiencies. Still, the work provided evidence of faster, better response/remission rates when pharmacogenetics are used to provide treatment of depression |

*Data from* Refs.[22,29–35]

**Table 2**
New directions for mental health in primary care

| Item/Definition | Current Status | Projected Impact |
|---|---|---|
| Measurement-based care (MBC)[36]<br>MBC seeks:<br>• Optimization, accuracy, and speed: patients receive most appropriate treatments and best possible results with least patient burden in a most economical way<br>• To attain correct diagnosis and management as often and in as timely manner as possible<br>• As compared with usual care, MBC more precisely defines problems through regular, targeted, assessment of key clinical outcomes informing an action plan | • Not standard clinical practice for mental health<br>• Existing gap between research/practice outcomes<br>• To implement MBC: establishment of clear expectations/guidelines<br>• Foster practice-based implementation capacities<br>• Change financial incentives<br>• Assist providers adopting to MBC<br>• Development/expansion of MBC science base<br>• Engagement of consumers/families<br>• Use of evidence-based screening/diagnostic instruments as a norm<br>• Pharmacogenetic testing/assays | Measurement-based care adopted as standard of care could transform psychiatric practice, moving mental health into the health care mainstream, improving quality of care, access, enhancing recovery time, and lower economic burden for patients with mental illness<br>• Examples: pharmacogenetic assays<br>• Use of evidence-informed screens and treatments<br>• Team approaches |
| Pharmacogenetic assays and updates[37] | Pharmacokinetic and/or pharmacodynamic assays determining individual genetic propensity for/against cytochrome P450 pathways, determining sense of particular medicine agent efficacy working optimally/sub-optimally/against genetic makeup.<br>• Medicare reimbursed<br>• Ease of use: Buccal swab<br>• Accuracy continues to develop<br>• Some firms update without added costs | • Savings of medication and indirect health care costs compared with those receiving treatment as usual<br>• Projected increase in quality-adjusted life-years of 0.316 y<br>• Evidence limited although used in practice |

| | | |
|---|---|---|
| Telehealth access[38] | Linking provider and patient through web-based means in an articulated agreement using agency to provide access for screen face-to-face encounters in which psychiatric mental health is provided.<br>Rapid growth:<br>• Driven by the increasing demand for mental health services<br>• Shortage/distribution of mental health providers<br>• Increasing technology availability<br>• Third-party reimbursement | Telemental health limits/opportunities:<br>• Access to care increased<br>• Multiple logistical demands can lead to link interruptions<br>• Some third-party payer limits<br>• Organizational approach/support/technology are key on both side of encounter<br>• Access increases care coordination<br>• 24/7 coverage<br>• Improve quality, equity, and affordability of depression management<br>• Patients increasingly request patient centered access to care |
| Wellness-based reimbursement incentive payment strategies[39] | • Medicare access/Children's Health Insurance Program (CHIP) Reauthorization<br>• Act of 2015 (Medicare Access and CHIP Reauthorization Act [MACRA]) a stepping stone for revised Part B Medicare payments<br>• Core aspect of this legislation with permanent repealing of Sustainable Growth Rate<br>• MACRA's Importance: key in development of new payment framework for health care delivery divided into the Merit-Based Incentive Payment System (MIPS)/ advanced alternative payment methods<br>• Introduced 2 y ago, in trial state to become mandatory at some point in near future<br>• Bonus incentive payments to be awarded to practices attaining wellness benchmarks<br>• Private payers historically follow Medicare dynamics | • Financial incentives for population wellness outcomes<br>• Increased provider satisfaction<br>• Confusion in the system relating to overhaul of payment system and the economic incentives based on the former/ current system.<br>• Encounter-based payments will be replaced by wellness, quality-based encounters, in time |

(continued on next page)

**Table 2**
*(continued)*

| Item/Definition | Current Status | Projected Impact |
|---|---|---|
| Integrative care model uptake[40,41] | • Integrative care, simply stated is where people can receive physical and mental wellness care in a setting/organization<br>• Positive uptake for recipients of care for depression in integrative care settings reported by Cochrane Review meta-analysis[42]<br>• Many levels of integrative care available<br>• Provides coordination of care, payer, and transportation issues<br>• Faces numerous challenges to fully fold into US health care services<br>• Serves persons, communities, and mental wellness with regard to substance use issues<br>• Both recipients of care and providers report increases in encounter satisfaction<br>• Reduction of hospitalizations<br>• Recovery and trauma<br>• Centered framework adoption | • Uptake of model increased since Affordable Care Act and commensurate funding structures.<br>• 70% of depression care is initiated and followed in primary care<br>• Integrated electronic health records are essential, reducing service gaps/information gaps<br>• Payer structuring is cumbersome but in progress |

*Data from Refs.[36–41]*

received as an acceptable outcome, which differs from other somatic pathologic conditions. Depression begets depression: as a pathologic condition, depression is not held in high esteem by providers (see Grue and colleagues);[27] being stigmatized, depression ranks 30 of 38 disease categories in prestige globally: possessing less stature in terms of disability, rather than a "serious disability" such as myocardial infarction and HIV. The disease state itself is not taken seriously, given its pervasive incidence and prevalence. Therefore "less than" full remission of symptoms is unfortunately the norm, and too often accepted as an acceptable outcome compared with other pathologic conditions.

## DISCUSSION

There are numerous barriers to effective management of depression in primary care that include the paucity of mental health providers, inadequately prepared providers, and the need for timely referrals to psychiatric providers when indicated. Current solutions include telemental health, measurement-based care, a Merit-Based Incentive Payment System, staff training, office-based consults/behavioral health provider(s), and integrative care model adoption.

The need for accurate differential diagnosis management pertinent to bipolar disorder includes lack of time for evidence-informed screens and thorough history taking because of varied presentations/co-morbidities. Differential diagnostics often result in diagnostic lateness of bipolarity and treatment of persons with bipolar affective disorders with antidepressant monotherapy leading to iatrogenic kindling mania risk. This can be addressed by appropriate screening and gathering of adequate history.

---

**Box 2**
**Clinical pearls**

Center for Medicare Systems in process of moving toward adoption of Merit-Based

Incentive Payment System (MIPS)[36] and wellness initiatives

Psychotherapy and psychopharmacology approaches combined yield; more robust results leading to recovery in insightful patients willing to participate[9]

All patients with depression recommended to be screened for bipolar disorder/other differentials[43]

Pediatric depression screening ages 12 to 17 years is recommended at every visit, can screen younger depending on development.[44] All adolescents to be screened for substance use at every encounter[42]

Women of childbearing/lactation age should be treated pharmacologically with the least teratogenic and/or harmful approaches, with reliable birth control in place, if sexually active when not family planning[22,45]

Screening of the elderly for depression at each encounter as a standard[46,47]

Using measurement-based instruments for efficient screening/diagnostics/treatments[36,39]

Where possible, use pharmacogenetic testing to reduce costs of time lost to efficacy[37]

Access care/providers via telemental health, use of telehealth consults, and/or face–to–face care via telehealth when face–to–face mental health provider(s) not accessible[38]

Integrative care models incorporate mental/physical wellness care within 1 organization, reducing service gaps due to relative accessibility[40–42]

*Data from* Refs.[9,22,36–47]

Other barriers include persistence of stigma related to mental health treatment, lack of psychoeducation for patients and providers, and time needed for a true cultural shift, which can take generations. However, the paradigm shift in primary delivery to wellness promoting Center for Medicare & Medicaid Services initiatives, rewarding wellness, rather than encounter volume, have initiated an industry disruption, but an essential culture shift among health care providers is needed. New treatment approaches for mental health in primary care are outlined in **Table 2**.

Depression is commonplace, most often recognized and treated in primary care[3] settings, by clinicians who may or may not be adequately prepared for its diverse presentations. Measurement-based practice promises assistance in more accurate diagnosis early on in presentations using treatment options based on evidence-informed practice. See **Box 2** for a review of current evidence-based clinical practice pearls.

## SUMMARY

Pharmacogenetic assays may speed recovery through introduction of more accurately targeted medicines. Moving into the future, avenues such as integrative care, telehealth, and wellness-based reimbursement incentives promise a welcome change to a landscape needing dynamic restructure and the mental health encounter environment in primary care.

## REFERENCES

1. World Health Organization. Depression and other common mental disorders: global health estimates. Geneva (Switzerland): World Health Organization; 2017. Available at: http://apps.who.int/iris/bitstream/handle/10665/254610/WHO-MSD-MER-2017.2-eng.pdf?sequence=1. Accessed November 11, 2018.
2. Pratt LA, Brody DJ. Depression in the U.S. household population, 2009-2012. NCHS Data Brief 2014;172:1–8. Available at: https://www.cdc.gov/nchs/data/databriefs/db172.htm. Accessed November 11, 2018.
3. Halverson J, Bienenfeld D, Bhalla R, et al. Depression clinical presentation: history, physical examination, major depressive disorder. 2018. Available at: Emedicine. medscape.com; https://emedicine.medscape.com/article/286759-clinical#showall. Accessed November, 24 2018.
4. World Health Organization. Depression. 2017. Available at: https://www.who.int/mental_health/management/depression/en/. Accessed November, 8 2018.
5. Mojtabai R, Olfson M, Han B. National trends in the prevalence and treatment of depression in adolescents and young adults. Pediatrics 2016;138(6):9.
6. World Health Organization. Adolescent mental health. 2018. Available at: http://www.who.int/mental_health/maternal-child/adolescent/en/. Accessed November, 15 2018.
7. Goldberg JS, Bell CE Jr, Pollard DA. Revisiting the monoamine hypothesis of depression: a new perspective. Perspect Medicin Chem 2014;6:1–8.
8. McEwen BS. Plasticity of the hippocampus: adaptation to chronic stress and allostatic load. Ann N Y Acad Sci 2001;933(1):265. Available at: https://libproxy.usouthal.edu/login?url=https://search.ebscohost.com/login.aspx?direct=true&db=edb&AN=91503744&site=eds-live.
9. Duman R. Pathophysiology of depression and innovative treatments: remodeling glutamatergic synaptic connections. Dialogues Clin Neurosci 2014;16(1):11–27. Available at: https://www-ncbi-nlm-nih-gov.libproxy.usouthal.edu/pubmed/24733968.
10. Sederer LI. The social determinants of mental health. Psychiatr Serv 2016;67(2):234–5.

11. Assari S. Social determinants of depression: the intersections of race, gender, and socioeconomic status. Brain Sci 2017;7(12). https://doi.org/10.3390/brainsci7120156.

12. Andermann A. Screening for social determinants of health in clinical care: moving from the margins to the mainstream. Public Health Rev 2018;39:19.

13. Rusner M, Berg M, Begley C. Bipolar disorder in pregnancy and childbirth: a systematic review of outcomes. BMC Pregnancy Childbirth 2016;16:331–72.

14. American Psychiatric Association. Diagnostic and statistical manual of mental disorders. 5th edition. Washington, DC: American Psychiatric Association; 2013.

15. SAMSHA-HRSA Center for Integrated Health Solutions. Screening tools. Available at: https://www.integration.samhsa.gov/clinical-practice/screening-tools. Accessed December 20, 2018.

16. US Preventive Services Task Force (nd.)PHQ-9. Available at: https://www.uspreventiveservicetaskforce.org/Home/GetFileByID218. Accessed November 30, 2018.

17. Prime MD. Prime-MD patient health questionnaire. Available at: http://www.oacbdd.org/clientuploads/Docs/2010/Spring%20Handouts/Session%20220j.pdf. Accessed November 30, 2018.

18. Bright futures (nd.) pediatric symptom checklist, instructions for use. Available at: https://wwwbrightfutures.org/mentalhealtyh/pdf/professionals/ped_symptom_chklst.pdf. Accessed November 30, 2018.

19. Posner K, Brent D, Lucas C, et al. Columbia-suicide severity rating scale. Columbia-suicide severity rating scale, pediatric-since last contact- communities and healthcare version 6/23/10. The Research Foundation for Mental Hygiene, Inc. Available at: https://cssrs.columbia.edu/wp-content/uploads/C-SSRS_Pediatric-SLC_11.14.16.pdf. Accessed November 30, 2018.

20. Megellan. Cage and Cage-AID introduction and scoring. Available at: https://docs.google.com/document/d/1_qwV9mb5BzHx1XZisGxCGTtOluh68L3y24B-C58AYbl/edit. Accessed November 30, 2018.

21. American Psychological Association. Beck depression inventory. 2018. Available at: https://www.apa.org/pi/about/publications/caregivers/practice-settings/assessment/tools/beck-depression.aspx. Accessed November 30, 2018.

22. Massachusetts General Hospital Center for Women's Mental Health Reproductive Psychiatry Resource & Information Center. Psychiatric disorders during pregnancy, weighing the risks and benefits of pharmacologic treatment during pregnancy. 2018. Available at: https://womensmentalhealth.org/specialty-clinics/psychiatric-disorders-during-pregnancy/. Accessed November 30, 2018.

23. Sage therapeutics. Using the edinburgh postnatal depression scale. 2018. Available at: https://www.knowppd.com/epds-ppd-screening/. Accessed November 30, 2018.

24. North American Menopause Society. Depression and menopause. 2018. Available at: https://www.menopause.org/for-women/menopauseflashes/mental-health-at-menopause/depression-menopause. Accessed November 30, 2018.

25. Greenberg S. The geriatric depression scale, revised 2012. Try this. Best practices in nursing care to older adults. 2019 Issue 4. Available at: https://consultgeri.org/try-this/general-assessment/issue-4.pdf. Accessed November 30, 2018.

26. Balsamo M, Cataldi F, Carlucci L, et al. Assessment of late-life depression via self-report measures: a review. Clin Interv Aging 2018;13:2021–44.

27. Grue J, Johannessen LE, Rasmussen EF. Prestige rankings of chronic diseases and disabilities. A survey among professionals in the disability field. Soc Sci Med 2015;124:180–6.

28. Fiske A, Wetherell JL, Gatz M. Depression in older adults. Annu Rev Clin Psychol 2009;5:363–89.
29. CDC. Suicide rates rising across the U.S. Comprehensive prevention goes beyond a focus on mental health concerns. CDC Newsroom. 2018. Available at: https://www.cdc.gov/media/releases/2018/p0607-suicide-prevention.html. Accessed November 30, 2018.
30. Zuckerbrot RA, Cheung A, Jensen PS, et al. Guidelines for Adolescent Depression in Primary Care (GLAD-PC): Part I. Practice preparation, identification, assessment, and initial management. Pediatrics 2018;141(3):1–21.
31. Moreland CS, Bonin L, Brent D, et al. Pediatric unipolar depression and pharmacotherapy: choosing a medication. UpToDate. The Netherlands: Wolters Kluwer; 2018. Available at: https://wwwuptodate-com.libproxy.usouthal.edu/contents/pediatric-unipolar-depression-andpharmacotherapy-choosing-a-medication?topicRef51231&source5see_link. Accessed November 26, 2018.
32. Tamburello AC, Kathpal A, Reeves R. Characteristics of inmates who misuse prescription medication. J Correct Health Care 2017;23(4):449–58.
33. Gers L, Petrovic M, Perkisas S, et al. Antidepressant use in older inpatients: current situation and application of the revised STOPP criteria. Ther Adv Drug Saf 2018;9(8):373–84.
34. By the American Geriatrics Society 2015 Beers Criteria Update Expert Panel. American Geriatrics Society 2015 updated beers criteria for potentially inappropriate medication use in older adults. J Am Geriatr Soc 2015;63(11):2227–46. Available at: https://www-ncbi-nlm-nih-gov.libproxy.usouthal.edu/pubmed/26446832.
35. Rosenblatt JD, Lee Y, McIntyre RS. The effect of pharmacogenomic testing on response and remission rates in the acute treatment of major depressive disorder: a meta-analysis. J Affect Disord 2018;241:484–91.
36. Harding KJ, Rush AJ, Arbuckle M, et al. Measurement-based care in psychiatric practice: a policy framework for implementation. J Clin Psychiatry 2011;72(8):1136–43.
37. Bousman CA, Hopwood M. Commercial pharmacogenetic-based decision-support tools in psychiatry. Lancet Psychiatry 2016;3(6):585–90.
38. Adams S, Rice MJ, Jones SL, et al. TeleMental health: standards, reimbursement, and interstate practice. J Am Psychiatr Nurses Assoc 2018;(4):295–305.
39. Hirsch JA, Rosenkrantz AB, Ansari SA, et al. Are you ready for MIPS? J Neurointerv Surg 2017;9:714–6.
40. SAMSHA-HRSA. Advancing behavioral health integration within NCQA recognized patient-centered homes. SAMSHA-HRSA Center for Integrated Health Services (online). Available at: https://www.integration.samhsa.gov/integrated-care-models. Accessed December 25, 2018.
41. SAMSHA-HRSA. Advancing behavioral health integration within NCQA recognized patient-centered homes. SAMSHA-HRSA national center for integrated health solutions. 2014. White Paper. Washington DC. Available at: https://docs.google.com/document/d/1lYmOBUsVDst_1zkcyglontUxfh47FQkkU9n9XbeYDJ4/edit#. Accessed Deccember 20, 2018.
42. Archer J, Bower P, Gilbody S, et al. Collaborative care for depression and anxiety problems. Cochrane Database Syst Rev 2012;(10):CD006525.
43. Tolliver BK, Anton RF. Assessment and treatment of mood disorders in the context of substance abuse. Dialogues Clin Neurosci 2015;17(2):181–90. Available at: https://www.ncbi.nlm.nih.gov/pubmed/26246792.
44. Knight J, Roberts T, Gabrielli J, et al. Adolescent alcohol and substance use and abuse. In: Tanski S, Garfunkel LC, Duncan PM, et al, editors. Performing

preventative services: a bright futures handbook. 3rd edition. Cherry Hill (NJ): American Academy of Pediatrics; 2010. p. 103. Ch. 55.
45. Bonham A. Why are 50 percent of pregnancies in the U.S. unplanned? Special edition, A Woman's nation changes everything. The Shriver Report 10.21 2013. Available at: http://shriverreport.org/why-are-50-percent-of-pregnancies-in-the-us-unplanned-adrienne-d-bonham/. Accessed November 15, 2018.
46. Miller J, Johnson SL, Eisner L. Assessment tools for adult bipolar disorder. Clin Psychol 2009;16(2):188–201.
47. Bosanquet K, Adamson J, Atherton K, et al. Collaborative care for Screen-Positive Elders with major depression (CASPER plus): a multicentered randomized controlled trial of clinical effectiveness and cost-effectiveness. Health Technol Assess 2017;21(67):1–252.

# Anxiety Disorders in Primary Care Settings

Ashley S. Love, DNP, PMHNP-BC[a],*, Rene Love, PhD, DNP, PMHNP-BC, FNAP[b]

## KEYWORDS

- Anxiety disorders • Primary care • Pharmacologic treatment

## KEY POINTS

- Anxiety disorders are the most common mental health disorders seen in primary care settings.
- Identification and treatment of anxiety disorders in primary care settings is difficult and often underdiagnosed due to lack of typical presentations and time constraints.
- Effective treatment of anxiety disorders can be improved with utilization of psychometric tools and pharmacologic treatment guidelines.

## BACKGROUND AND SIGNIFICANCE

Anxiety disorders are the most common mental health disorders in the United States and one of the most common mental health problems seen in general medical settings.[1] Lifetime prevalence of anxiety is estimated to be as high as 29% in the United States.[2] However, identification and treatment of anxiety disorders are often difficult in general medical settings. The lack of common presentations with anxiety disorders and time constraints in the clinic setting pose challenges for medical providers within the primary care setting. Results from one study show these rates of misdiagnosis to be as high as 71% for generalized anxiety disorder (GAD).[3] When anxiety is left untreated, societal costs are substantive. In the United States, societal costs of anxiety disorders are estimated to be more than $48 billion per year.[4] Adults with untreated social anxiety disorders miss on average 24.7 days of work per year due to the diagnosis.[5] Given the significance of health care costs, decreased quality of

The authors whose names are listed certify that they have no affiliations with or involvement in any organization or entity with any financial interest (such as honoraria; educational grants; participation in speakers' bureaus; membership, employment, consultancies, stock ownership, or other equity interest; and expert testimony or patent-licensing arrangements) or nonfinancial interest (such as personal or professional relationships, affiliations, knowledge, or beliefs) in the subject matter or materials discussed in this article.

[a] Serenity Psychiatric Care, Benson Health Clinic, 66 Club Road, Suite 140, Eugene, OR 97401, USA; [b] University of Arizona, College of Nursing, 1305 N Martin Avenue, PO Box 210203, Tucson, AZ 85721-0203, USA
* Corresponding author.
E-mail address: alove@serenitypsychiatriccare.org

life, and loss of workforce productivity for patients with anxiety disorders, it is imperative that medical settings understand how to properly identify, diagnose, and treat these disorders.

## PATHOGENESIS OF ANXIETY DISORDERS

Multiple factors have been targeted for the development of GAD; however, most researchers agree that the cause is epigenetic in nature.[6] Genetic studies of the development of anxiety disorders have found heritability estimates between 20% and 65%, with the earlier the onset of symptoms, the higher the likelihood of a genetic component.[7] Research in both animal and human studies have found the cortico-amygdala circuitry system to have an important role in anxiety disorders, specifically, the hippocampus, prefrontal cortex, and dorsal anterior cingulate cortex.[8,9] Gene analysis and neuroimaging studies have found positive associations between the serotonin transporter gene (5-HTT) and the catechol-O-methyltransferase.[8,10]

The other 35% to 80% of factors are caused by environmental factors, including stressful life events, traumatic experiences, disrupted attachments, and parental emotional problems.[6] Parenting styles and modeling can play significant roles in the development of anxiety disorders, especially, those parents who exhibit anxious, overly critical, insensitive, or overprotective parenting behaviors.[11] Other ways in which children learn anxious or fearful responses from their environment include direct negative experiences (neglect, abuse), false alarms (perceiving a situation negatively with no evidence to support this believe), and/or vicariously witnessing or being told something is dangerous.[8]

## ASSESSMENT

Patients with anxiety disorders are 2 times more likely than the general population to present initially with somatic complaints.[12] These complaints range from one specific distressing symptom, such as diarrhea or insomnia, to numerous seemingly unrelated symptoms. Common presenting somatic complaints include palpitations, diaphoresis, nausea, abdominal distress, dizziness, and restlessness.[13] Symptoms that have been medically worked up with no identified cause should warrant further assessment to rule out anxiety disorders. **Table 1** provides an overview of common symptoms and characteristics of anxiety disorders.

## GENERALIZED ANXIETY DISORDER

GAD is defined as excessive, uncontrolled worry and tension about daily events and activities occurring more days than not for at least 6 months. GAD occurs when the worries are persistent and cause notable impairments in day-to-day life. Typical symptoms include irritability, fatigue, restlessness, sleep disturbances, and muscle tension.[14] It is considered a chronic illness with symptom severity waxing and waning; however, remittance of symptoms is possible with proper identification and treatment.[15]

### Children and Adolescents

Anxiety disorders are the most common childhood onset of psychiatric disorders[8] affecting between 2.9% and 4.6% of children and adolescents.[14] In childhood, distribution tends to be equal for both women and men; however, in adolescents the female-to-male ratio is as high as 6:1.[8] Initial onset of symptoms occurs in school age years with typical onset around 7 years old.[8]

| Table 1 |
| --- |
| **Comparison of anxiety disorders** |

| Anxiety Disorder | Key Characteristics |
| --- | --- |
| Generalized Anxiety Disorder | Persistent and extreme worry, stress, and anxiety about day-to-day life events |
| Social Anxiety Disorder | Excessive fear and worry around everyday interactions and social situations specifically with how one is perceived and judged by others |
| Posttraumatic Stress Disorder | Persistent fear or emotional distress as a result of injury or severe psychological shock to a traumatic event with ongoing intrusive symptoms related to the event |
| Obsessive Compulsive Disorder | Persistent, uncontrollable thoughts (obsessions) that cause fear, anxiety, and emotional distress. Obsessions are commonly accompanied by behaviors (compulsions) that are done to mitigate the anxiety and fear caused by the obsessions |
| Panic Disorder | Characterized by reoccurring panic attacks or sudden feelings of terror and discomfort that arise within minutes |

*Data from* American Psychiatric Association. Diagnostic and Statistical Manual of Mental Disorders. 5th ed. Arlington, VA: American Psychiatric Association; 2013.

Presentation of symptoms in both children and adolescents typically focus around fears about the family (health-related and safety concerns) and/or school performance. The symptoms are difficult to stop and/or control. These preoccupations tend to manifest in an "all or nothing" cognitive bias and perfectionism. If the child does not perform perfectly, they develop thoughts and feelings of negative self-worth (ie, they are no good). Rather than focusing on their successes, they tend to perseverate on their mistakes. Many of these children and adolescents have complaints of decreased sleep as a result; however, other clinical manifestations include somatic symptoms such as headaches, decreased appetite, and stomach aches, excessive need for reassurance, explosiveness and oppositional behavior, and/or avoidance.[8]

## Adults

GAD is the most common anxiety disorder in primary care settings. It is estimated that 15% to 20% of patients meet criteria for anxiety disorders in primary care settings.[16] Lifetime prevalence of GAD has been shown to be up to 33.7% of the general population.[17] Women are twice as likely as men to have GAD.[17]

Although persistent worrying is considered the basis for GAD, most patients present with other symptoms related to autonomic hyperactivity, hyperarousal, and muscle tension. Many of these patients have complaints of fatigue, poor sleep, difficulty relaxing, and somatic symptoms including headache and pain in back, shoulders, and neck areas. Younger adults tend to present with greater severity of symptoms than older adults and with more autonomic anxiety.[14,18] Older adult worries tend to revolve around physical independence and physical health.[18]

Predictors of GAD include the following:

- Chronic physical illnesses,
- Comorbid psychiatric diagnosis (depression, phobias, past history of GAD),
- Recent adverse life events,
- Poverty,
- Female gender,

- Parental loss,
- History of mental problems in parents, and
- Low affective support during childhood.[15]

## SOCIAL ANXIETY DISORDER

Social anxiety disorder is characterized by excessive fear and worry over being scrutinized, embarrassed, and/or humiliated in social settings.[14] There are no significant differences in degree of impairment between lower-, middle-, and higher-income groups.[5] Untreated, social anxiety disorder often leads to the development of major depression, substance abuse, and/or other mental health problems.[19]

### Children and Adolescents

Social anxiety disorder commonly presents in childhood or adolescence.[19] The average age of onset in the United States is 13 years.[5]

Typically, children and adolescents present with social anxiety in events or settings that involve peers or adults who are less familial. Children may exhibit symptoms such as crying, freezing, clinging, avoiding speaking, or tantrums. During the assessment interview, children and adolescents will generally be shy or withdrawn with minimal eye contact or responses to questions until they have had time to develop a rapport with the clinician. They will often describe fears of being laughed at, embarrassed, and/or of saying or doing the wrong thing. Their worries tend to revolve around what others think of them rather than what they think of themselves.[20]

### Adults

Social anxiety disorder affects between 3% and 7% of adults in the United States per year; however, lifetime prevalence rates are as high as 12%.[19] Lifetime risks of social anxiety disorder are associated with the following risk factors:

- Age of onset,
- Female gender,
- Unemployment,
- Unmarried (never married or widowed/separated/divorced),
- Lower educational status, and
- Low household income.[5]

In social or performance situations, symptoms of social anxiety disorder in adults include physical manifestations of anxiety such as diaphoresis, tremors, heart palpitations, and facial flushing, which can sometimes result in a panic attack. The person will often worry for hours or days before the feared event or setting; however, there is commonly a fear that others will notice their irrational anxiety and thus symptoms may go unnoticed. They may even avoid the feared setting or event entirely, or if they participate, it is with immense anxiety or more subtle avoidance behaviors such as poor eye contact and/or not engaging in conversations with others. Common feared events and situations include public speaking, large crowds, eating or drinking in public, or even using a public urinal. After the event is over, the person may perseverate on their shortcomings, feel depressed, and berate themselves.[19]

## POSTTRAUMATIC STRESS DISORDER

Posttraumatic stress disorder (PTSD) presents with 4 main symptom clusters: intrusion, avoidance, negative alterations in mood and cognition, and hyperarousal.[14] To distinguish PTSD from other anxiety disorders, those with the diagnosis must have an event precipitating the symptoms. The reoccurring and uncontrollable thoughts, dreams, and emotional reactions are related to the traumatic event. In some individuals, dissociative reactions can be present to the extent that the person feels they are reliving the event and may be unaware of their present surroundings.[14]

Individual prerisk factors for the development of PTSD include the following:

- Female gender,
- Lower education,
- Lower socioeconomic status,
- Previous trauma,
- Age at trauma,
- Childhood adversity,
- Personal and/or family psychiatric history,
- History of child abuse,
- Poor social support, and
- Initial severity of reaction to the traumatic event.[21]

### Children and Adolescents

Although more than 60% of children and adolescence will experience some sort of traumatic event before adulthood, only about 15.9% will develop PTSD.[22,23] Rates are similar between boys and girls; however, boys are more likely to experience physical violence, whereas girls are more likely to be victims of sexual abuse.[24] Those who experienced the trauma in childhood have more difficulty with affect regulation with an increased severity of symptoms.[23]

In children, nightmares are not always directly related to the traumatic event but can cause sleep difficulties, including a fear of awakening during or after the dream. Negative emotions in children also increase, including fear, guilt, anger, and shame. Emotional reactivity increases and can present as symptoms of irritability, anger outbursts, physical violence, or temper tantrums. In addition, anhedonia, decreased concentration, and decreased social connectedness to others can result in the child or adolescent feeling detached or estranged.[23]

### Adults

The lifetime prevalence of PTSD ranges from 6.1% to 9.2% with higher rates found in North American countries than other regions worldwide.[5] Women are twice as likely to develop symptoms of PTSD after a traumatic event.[21]

Symptoms of PTSD are most often triggered by responses to trauma-related stimuli leading to flashbacks, anxiety, and fleeing or combative behavior. These individuals typically try to avoid the trauma-related stimuli to reduce this intense arousal; however, this can result in anhedonia, emotional numbing, and even detachment from others.

## OBSESSIVE COMPULSIVE DISORDER

Obsessive compulsive disorder (OCD) is characterized by uncontrollable, reoccurring thoughts, sensations, feelings (obsessions), behaviors that drive them to do something repeatedly (compulsions), or both. The individual can attempt to ignore or suppress the obsessive thoughts or to neutralize them by some other thought or action, such as performing a compulsion. Compulsive behaviors then are aimed at reducing anxiety or preventing some imagined event or situation; however, these acts are excessive and/or not realistically connected to what they are designed to neutralize.[14]

Compulsions are not pleasurable for the individual and thus not to be mistaken for an impulsive act that is associated with immediate gratification (ie, gambling, shopping). Obsessions are also not associated with day-to-day worries, which occur in GAD or are regarding perceived defects in physical appearance, which occur in body dysmorphicdisorder.[25]

### Children and Adolescents

OCD typically presents in childhood or adolescence and persists throughout a person's life. Without treatment, symptoms are chronic but fluctuate for most individuals. Average onset of symptoms is between 9 and 11 years for male children and 11 and 13 years for female children. Mens are more commonly affected in childhood than women.[26]

Children with OCD are more likely to present with obvious compulsions than with obsessions such as the washing of their hands excessively. For some children, detecting obsessions can be difficult for practitioners because very young children may not be able to verbally describe their obsessions. Untreated and undiagnosed OCD in children and adolescents can lead to difficulty with separation-individuation from parents and occupational achievement as adults.[27]

Rarely, children may develop sudden onset of episodic symptoms with concomitant motor tics, hyperactivity, or choreiform movements. This presentation has been associated with underlying infectious agents in several case studies of children with OCD.[28]

### Adults

The lifetime prevalence rate of OCD among adults in North America is estimated at 3.7%.[29] Although the specific content of compulsions and obsessions varies among individuals, there are identifiable themes, or "symptom dimensions," which include the following:

- Harm: examples include fears of harm to self or others and associated checking compulsions (eg, door locks)
- Symmetry: examples include alignment or symmetry obsessions and counting, ordering, and repeating compulsions
- Cleaning: examples include fear of contamination and cleaning compulsions (eg, excessive hand washing)
- Forbidden or unacceptable thoughts: examples include sexual, religious, and/or aggressive obsessions and related compulsions[30]

Because of the severity of symptoms, it is common for adults with OCD to exhibit avoiding behaviors and struggle with suicidal ideation.[30] Beliefs around obsessions and compulsions can cause individuals to have dysfunctional beliefs including perfectionism, overvaluing need to control thoughts and their importance, and a tendency to overestimate threats.

### PANIC DISORDER

Individuals with panic disorder suffer from reoccurring panic attacks that are either unexpected or triggered by something in their environment. Panic attacks are short episodes of intense fear that culminate within minutes. Symptoms of panic attacks include the following:

- Feelings of impending doom,
- Trembling or shaking,

- Paresthesias,
- Diaphoresis,
- Heart palpitations, accelerated heart rate, or pounding heartbeat,
- Sensations of choking, shortness of breath, chest pain, or not being able to catch one's breath, and
- Feelings of being out of control.[31]

People with panic attacks often worry about when the next episode will occur and will actively try to avoid a reoccurrence of a panic attack by avoiding things, places, or behaviors that they associate with panic attacks.[31] Concern over upcoming panic attacks causes significant disruption in a person's life and can lead to the development of other psychological disorders such as agoraphobia.[31]

### Children and Adolescents

Rarely do panic attacks begin in childhood or adolescence, but when they do, they can be extremely debilitating for the individual.[32] Without recognition and appropriate treatment, panic attacks can interfere with the child or adolescent's schoolwork, development, and relationships. Since the fear of panic attacks can lead to anxiety even when panic attacks are not present, the child or adolescent's mood is also affected. Some children and adolescents with panic disorder can develop depression and suicidal thoughts/behaviors and are at higher risk of abusing drugs or alcohol.[32]

### Adults

Statistics on lifetime prevalence rates of panic attacks for adults for all countries combined has been shown to be around 13.2%.[5] Panic attacks typically develop after age 20 years with the median age of onset being 32 years with higher prevalence in women.[5] They can lead to interruptions in one's occupational and social life, as it is common for those with panic attacks to miss work and avoid situations where a panic attack might occur. It can also be a financial burden for those experiencing panic attacks, as they tend to have more frequent visits to their doctor and/or emergency room, convinced that they are experiencing a life-threatening medical emergency.[33]

## PSYCHOMETRIC SCREENING TOOLS
### Children and Adolescents

Some studies suggest that parents and children can differ in their reports on symptoms and severity; therefore, it is pertinent to obtain the child or adolescent's own perception of symptoms.[34] Some children may even feel more comfortable endorsing symptoms of anxiety and related functional impairments in a questionnaire versus in an interview.[35] For an overview of free child and adolescent psychometric scales for anxiety see **Table 2**.

### Adults

Because of time constraints in primary care settings, psychometric tools can be helpful in identifying anxiety disorders in adult populations. Psychometric tools assist the provider in diagnosing, treating, and assessing changes in anxiety levels following treatment response; however, it is pertinent to ensure that the patient's subjective response is also considered when evaluating changes in symptoms severity. Treatment decisions should thus be dictated by patient choice and subjective experience.[4] For an overview of free adult psychometric scales for anxiety see **Table 3**.

**Table 2**
Free, online child and adolescent psychometric scales for anxiety disorders

| Scale | Description | Number of Items | Administration | Psychometric Properties | Obtainable |
|---|---|---|---|---|---|
| Children Yale-Brown Obsessive Compulsive Scale (CY-BOCS) | Screening tool for obsessive compulsive behaviors Monitors symptom changes over time | 10 | Parent-reported | Sensitive to change | http://icahn.mssm.edu/research/centers/center-of-excellence-for-ocd/rating-scales |
| Penn State Worry Questionnaire for Children (PSWQ-C) | Screening tool for generalized anxiety disorder | 16 | Self-reported | | http://www.childfirst.ucla.edu/Resources.html |
| Child PTSD Symptom Scale (CPSS) | Screening and diagnostic tool for children and adolescents aged 8–18 y | 24 | Self-administered or clinician-reported | Sensitive to change | ude.nnepu.dem.liam@aof |
| Mini-Social Phobia Inventory (Mini-SPIN)-1 | Screening tool for social phobia studied in adolescents | 3 | Self-administered | Accurate and efficacious | david011@mc.duke.edu |
| Hamilton Rating Scale for Anxiety (HAM-A)- | Screening tool for anxiety symptoms studied in adolescents Monitors symptom changes over time | 14 | Clinician-reported | Sensitive to change | http://psychology-tools.com/hamilton-anxiety-rating-scale/ |

*Data from* Beidas RS, Stewart RB, Walsh L, et. al. Free, brief, and validated: Standardized instruments for low-resource mental health settings. *Cogn Behav Pract.* 2016; 22(1):5-19 and Connor KM, Kobak KA, Churchill LE, et. al. Mini-SPIN: a brief screening assessment for generalized social anxiety disorder. Depress. Anxiety 2001; 14(2):137-140.

**Table 3**
Free, online adult psychometric scales for anxiety disorders

| Measure | Description | Number of Items | Administration | Psychometric Properties | Obtainable |
|---|---|---|---|---|---|
| Generalized Anxiety Disorder Screener (GAD-7) | Screening and diagnostic tool for generalized anxiety disorder Monitors symptom changes over time | 7 | Self-administered | Reliability in primary care settings was 0.91 | https://www.integration.samhsa.gov/clinical-practice/screening-tools#anxiety |
| Penn State Worry Questionnaire (PSWQ) | Screening tool for generalized anxiety disorder Differentiates PTSD from generalized anxiety disorder | 16 | Self-administered | 71.7% sensitivity and 99.9% specificity | https://www.outcometracker.org/library/PSWQ.pdf |
| Hamilton Rating Scale for Anxiety (HAM-A) | Screening tool for anxiety symptoms Monitors symptom changes over time | 14 | Clinician-reported | Sensitive to change | http://psychology-tools.com/hamilton-anxiety-rating-scale/ |
| Liebowitz Social Anxiety Scale Clinician/Self-Report (LSAS-CR/SR) | Assesses avoidance and fear of social situations Screening tool for social anxiety symptoms Monitors symptom changes overtime | 24 | Self-administered or clinician-reported | Sensitive to change | http://healthnet.umassmed.edu/mhealth/LiebowitzSocialAnxietyScale.pdf http://asp.cumc.columbia.edu/SAD/ |
| Social Phobia Inventory (SPIN) | Screening tool for social phobia Monitors symptom changes over time | 17 | Self-administered | Sensitive to change | http://www.psychtoolkit.com |
| Panic Disorder Severity Scale (PDSS) | Diagnostic and screening tool for Panic Disorder Monitors symptom changes over time | 7 | Clinician-reported | Sensitive to change | http://www.outcometracker.org |
| The PTSD Checklist–Civilian Version (PCL-C) | Diagnostic and screening tool for PTSD | 17 | Self-administered | Sensitive to change | http://www.istss.org/assessing-trauma/posttraumatic-stress-disorder-checklist.aspx |

*Data from Refs.*[36–38]

## PHARMACOTHERAPY

The major neurotransmitters studied in relation to the pharmacologic treatment of anxiety disorders include norepinephrine, serotonin, and gamma-aminobutyric acid. People with anxiety disorders have malfunctioning noradrenergic systems with low threshold levels for arousal. When coupled with an unpredictable increase in activity, anxiety symptoms manifest.[39]

The goal of medication treatment of anxiety is to reduce severity of symptoms, improve overall functioning, and attain remission of symptoms. There are numerous classes of anxiolytic medications that are approved for treatment of anxiety disorders; however, there are few studies directly comparing the efficacy of specific medications. Therefore, when selecting a medication, it is pertinent to consider patient preferences, severity of symptoms, comorbidities including past or current history of substance abuse, history of previous treatment, and cost.[13] It is always crucial to weigh the risks of pharmacologic treatment, but this is especially crucial in the child and adolescent populations due to concerns around increased risk of suicide with certain classes of medications.[40] Once a medication has been selected, it should be continued for 6 to 12 months after remission of symptoms to reduce likelihood of relapse.[40] **Tables 4** and **5** include an overview of pharmacologic treatment options for each anxiety disorder in children and adolescents and adults, respectively, including common side effects, dosage range, and approvals from Food and Drug Administration.

## NONPHARMACOLOGIC STRATEGIES

Psychotherapy modalities and interventions have been widely explored in the treatment of anxiety disorders. Among these different therapies, cognitive behavioral therapy (CBT) has the strongest evidence and is considered a first-line treatment option as monotherapy and/or concomitantly with medication treatment.[13] A combination of CBT with pharmacotherapy has been shown in several studies to be the superior choice in the treatment of children, adolescence, and older adults.[41,42] If accessibility or affordability is a concern, several studies have found that internet-based CBT for panic disorder, OCD, and PTSD are superior to placebo, placement on a waiting list, and results to be equivalent to standard CBT.[43]

Evidence supports that both short- and long-term exercises can have anxiolytic effects.[43,44] Adults who regularly exercise report experiencing fewer anxiety symptoms, supporting the assumption that exercise has protective factors against the development of psychological disorders.[45]

Another practice associated with anxiolytic effects is meditation.[46] Single mindfulness sessions, even as short as 5 minutes, offer psychological benefits including an increased sense of well-being and reduced anxiety levels.[47,48] When combined with aerobic exercise, either before or after, mindfulness may achieve higher additional anxiolytic benefits than exercise or medication alone.[49]

## DISCUSSION

Identification, treatment, and management of anxiety disorders can be challenging. Screening tools can be very helpful in recognizing symptoms of anxiety disorders so that further evaluation and work-up can be performed by the provider during the interview. The primary care provider is often the first to learn of a patient's anxiety or traumatic experience. More severe or treatment-resistant anxiety disorders are best managed with collaboration and consultation with mental health providers and therapists. In addition, referrals should be considered when there are multiple mental

**Table 4**
**Pharmacological treatment of anxiety disorder in children and adolescents**

| Medication | Dosage Range | Common Side Effects | Commonly Prescribed for (Bold for FDA Approval) | Comments |
|---|---|---|---|---|
| SSRI | | Nausea, insomnia, somnolence, jitteriness, diarrhea, sexual dysfunction | | Antidepressants increase the risk of suicidal thinking and behavior in children, adolescents, and young adults (18–24 y of age) with major depressive disorder (MDD) and other psychiatric disorders. |
| Citalopram | 10–40 mg | | OCD | |
| Fluoxetine | 7–18 y: 10–60 mg | | OCD | |
| Fluvoxamine | 8–11 y: IR: 25–200 mg
12–18 y: IR: 25–300 mg | | OCD | Note: When total daily dose of immediate release exceeds 50 mg, the dose should be given in 2 divided doses with larger portion administered at bedtime. The extended-release formulation has not been evaluated in pediatric patients. |
| Paroxetine | 7–17 y: 10–60 mg
8–17 y: 10–50 mg | | OCD
SAD | |
| Sertraline | 6–12 y: 25–200 mg
12–18 y: 50–200 mg | | OCD | |
| SNRI | | Nausea, insomnia, somnolence, jitteriness, sexual dysfunction, hypertension | | Antidepressants increase the risk of suicidal thinking and behavior in children, adolescents, and young adults (18–24 y of age) with MDD and other psychiatric disorders |
| Duloxetine | 7–17 y: 30–120 mg | | GAD | |
| Benzodiazepines | | Somnolence, dizziness | | Safety and efficacy not established in children and adolescents; however, used often but at lower end of dosing scale.
Use with caution due to risk of tolerance, abuse, addiction, overdose, and/or withdrawal symptoms. Must be discontinued gradually, as abrupt or overly rapid reduction can cause life-threatening withdrawal symptoms (ie, seizures). |

*(continued on next page)*

**Table 4**
*(continued)*

| Medication | Dosage Range | Common Side Effects | Commonly Prescribed for (Bold for FDA Approval) | Comments |
|---|---|---|---|---|
| Alprazolam | 7–18 y: IR: 0.005 mg/kg/dose or 0.125 mg/dose TID–0.02 mg/kg/dose or 0.06 mg/kg/d | | Anxiety | |
| Lorazepam | <12 y: 0.05 mg/kg/dose or 0.02–0.1 mg/kg/dose 12–18 y: 0.25–6 mg/d; maximum dose: 2 mg/dose | | Anxiety, acute | |
| Tricyclic Antidepressants | | Orthostasis, anticholinergic, weight gain, cardiac arrhythmias | | Use with caution in those with active suicidal ideation. May be lethal in overdose. Antidepressants increase the risk of suicidal thinking and behavior in children, adolescents, and young adults (18–24 y of age) with MDD and other psychiatric disorders |
| Clomipramine | 25–200 mg/d or 3 mg/kg/d | | OCD | Initially titrate in divided doses. After titration may give as single dose daily at bedtime. |
| Other medication | | | | |
| Hydroxyzine | <6 y: 50 mg/d 6–18 y: 50–100 mg/d | Dry mouth, dry eyes, sedation | **Anxiety, acute** | Usually administered in divided doses |

*Abbreviations:* IR, instant release; SNRI, serotonin-norepinephrine reuptake inhibitors; SSRI, selective serotonin reuptake inhibitors.

*Data from* Albano AM, Alvarez E, Brent D, et al. Psychotherapy for anxiety disorders in children and adolescents. https://www.uptodate.com/contents/psychotherapy-for-anxiety-disorders-in-children-and-adolescents. Updated December 4, 2018 and Stahl SM. *Prescriber's Guide.* 6th ed. Cambridge, UK: Cambridge University Press; 2017.

**Table 5**
Pharmacologic treatment of anxiety disorder in adults

| Medication | Dosage Range | Common Side Effects | Commonly Prescribed for (Bold for FDA Approval) | Comments |
|---|---|---|---|---|
| SSRI | | Nausea, insomnia, somnolence, jitteriness, diarrhea, sexual dysfunction | | First-line treatment of ongoing anxiety disorders<br>Antidepressants increase the risk of suicidal thinking and behavior in children, adolescents, and young adults (18–24 y of age) with major depressive disorder (MDD) and other psychiatric disorders |
| Citalopram | 10–40 mg/d<br>20–40 mg/d<br>10–40 mg/d<br>20–40 mg/d<br>20–40 mg/d | | GAD<br>OCD<br>Panic disorder<br>PTSD<br>SAD | Recommended maximum dosage is 40 mg due to concerns of QT prolongation<br>Contraindications: use of MAO inhibitors intended to treat psychiatric disorders (concurrently or within 14 d of discontinuing either citalopram or the MAO inhibitor [MAOI]); initiation of citalopram in a patient receiving linezolid or intravenous methylene blue; concomitant use with pimozide |
| Escitalopram | 10–20 mg/d<br>10–40 mg/d<br>5–20 mg/d<br>10–40 mg/d | | **GAD**<br>OCD<br>Panic disorder<br>PTSD | Contraindications: use of MAOIs intended to treat psychiatric disorders (concurrently or within 14 d of discontinuing either escitalopram or the MAOI); initiation of escitalopram in a patient receiving linezolid or intravenous methylene blue; concurrent use of pimozide |
| Fluoxetine | 20–80 mg/d<br>5–60 mg/d<br>10–80 mg/d<br>10–60 mg/d | | **OCD**<br>**Panic disorder**<br>PTSD<br>SAD | Contraindications: use of MAOIs intended to treat psychiatric disorders (concurrently, within 5 wk of discontinuing fluoxetine or within 2 wk of discontinuing the MAOI); initiation of fluoxetine in a patient receiving linezolid or intravenous methylene blue; use with pimozide or thioridazine |

(continued on next page)

**Table 5**
*(continued)*

| Medication | Dosage Range | Common Side Effects | Commonly Prescribed for (Bold for FDA Approval) | Comments |
|---|---|---|---|---|
| Fluvoxamine | IR: 50–300 mg/d<br>ER: 100–300 mg/d<br>IR: 25–200 mg/d<br>IR: 75 mg BID/d<br>IR: 50–300 mg/d<br>ER: 100–300 mg/d | | **OCD**<br>Panic disorder<br>PTSD<br>SAD | Note: manufacturer's labeling recommends that daily doses >100 mg be given in 2 divided doses, with the larger dose administered at bedtime<br>Contraindications: concurrent use with alosetron, pimozide, thioridazine, or tizanidine; use of MAOIs intended to treat psychiatric disorders (concurrently or within 14 d of discontinuing either fluvoxamine or the MAOI); initiation of fluvoxamine in a patient receiving linezolid or intravenous methylene blue |
| Paroxetine | 20–50 mg/d<br>20–60 mg/d<br>10–60 mg/d<br>CR: 12.5–75 mg/d<br>20–50 mg/d<br>20–60 mg/d<br>CR: 12.5–37.5 mg/d | | **GAD**<br>**OCD**<br>**Panic disorder**<br>**PTSD**<br>**SAD** | Contraindications: concurrent use with or within 14 d of MAOIs intended to treat psychiatric disorders; initiation in patients being treated with linezolid or methylene blue IV; concomitant use with pimozide or thioridazine; pregnancy (Brisdelle only) |
| Sertraline | 25–200 mg/d<br>50–200 mg/d<br>25–200 mg/d<br>25–200 mg/d<br>25–200 mg/d | | **GAD**<br>**OCD**<br>**Panic disorder**<br>**PTSD**<br>**SAD** | Contraindications: use of MAOIs including linezolid or methylene blue (concurrently or within 14 d of stopping an MAOI or sertraline); concurrent use with disulfiram (oral solution only); concurrent use with pimozide |
| SNRI | | Nausea, insomnia, somnolence, jitteriness, sexual dysfunction, hypertension | | Second-line treatment for ongoing anxiety disorders<br>Antidepressants increase the risk of suicidal thinking and behavior in children, adolescents, and young adults (18–24 y of age) with MDD and other psychiatric disorders<br>Contraindications: use of MAOIs intended to treat psychiatric disorders (concurrently or within 14 d of discontinuing the MAOI); initiation of MAOI intended to treat psychiatric disorders within 7 d of discontinuing venlafaxine; initiation in patients receiving linezolid or IV methylene blue |

| Drug | Dosage | Indications | Adverse effects | Comments |
|---|---|---|---|---|
| Duloxetine | 30-120 mg/d | **GAD** | | |
| Venlafaxine | ER: 37.5–225 mg/d<br>IR: 75 mg TID–350 mg/d<br>ER: 75–350 mg/d<br>ER: 37.5–225 mg/d<br>ER: 37.5–300 mg/d<br>ER: 37.5–225 mg/d | **GAD**<br>**OCD**<br>**Panic disorder**<br>**PTSD**<br>**SAD** | | |
| Benzodiazepines | | | Somnolence, dizziness | Lowest possible effective dose for shortest possible period of time<br>Usually administered in divided doses<br>Use with caution due to risk of tolerance, abuse, addiction, overdose, and/or withdrawal symptoms<br>Must be discontinued gradually, as abrupt or overly rapid reduction can cause life-threatening withdrawal symptoms (ie, seizures)<br>Contraindications: acute narrow-angle glaucoma; severe respiratory insufficiency (except during mechanical ventilation) |
| Alprazolam | IR: 0.25–4 mg/d<br>IR: 0.5–6 mg/d<br>ER: 0.5–6 mg/d | **GAD**<br>**Panic disorder** | | |
| Clonazepam | 0.25 BID–4 mg/d | **Panic disorder** | | |
| Diazepam | 2–40 mg/d | Anxiety disorder and symptoms of anxiety (short-term) | | |
| Lorazepam | 2–10 mg/d | Anxiety disorder | | |

*(continued on next page)*

**Table 5**
*(continued)*

| Medication | Dosage Range | Common Side Effects | Commonly Prescribed for (*Bold for FDA Approval*) | Comments |
|---|---|---|---|---|
| Tricyclic Antidepressants | | Orthostasis, anticholinergic, weight gain, cardiac arrhythmias | | Use with caution in those with active suicidal ideation. May be lethal in overdose **Antidepressants increase the risk of suicidal thinking and behavior in children, adolescents, and young adults (18–24 y of age) with MDD and other psychiatric disorders** Contraindications: acute recovery period after a myocardial infarction; use of MAOIs intended to treat psychiatric disorders (concurrently or within 14 d of discontinuing either imipramine or the MAOI) |
| Clomipramine | 25–250 mg/d 10–250 mg/d | | OCD Panic disorder | Initially titrate in divided doses. After titration may give as single dose daily at bedtime |
| Imipramine | 10–239 mg/d 50–300 mg/d | | Panic disorder PTSD | |
| Other medication | | | | |
| Buspirone | 10–30 mg/d in 2–3 divided doses; maximum 60 mg/d | Dizziness, seating, nausea, insomnia, somnolence | GAD | Administered in 2–3 divided doses Contraindications: concomitant use of MAOI or MAOI use within past 14 d before starting medication |

| | Dose | Side effects | Anxiety, acute | Notes |
|---|---|---|---|---|
| Hydroxyzine | 50–400 mg/d | Dry mouth, dry eyes, sedation | | Usually administered in divided doses Contraindications: prolonged QT interval, early pregnancy |
| Gabapentin | 300 mg BID–1800 mg TID; maximum 3600 mg/d 300 mg BID–1800 mg TID; maximum 3600 mg/d | Somnolence, dizziness | Anxiety (adjunct) SAD | Usually administered in divided doses |
| Pregabalin | IR: 150 mg BID–300 mg BID; maximum 600 mg/d 300 mg/d in 3 divided doses–600 mg/d | Somnolence, dizziness | GAD SAD | Usually administered in divided doses |
| Propranolol | 10–60 mg per anxiety-inducing event 10–240 mg/d | Bradycardia, hypotension, dizziness, weight gain | Anxiety, acute (SAD, performance anxiety, panic) PTSD, prophylactic | Encourage patient to try out medication before precipitating event to determine tolerability and efficacy May theoretically block effects of stress from trauma but evidence is limited and mixed Contraindications: history of asthma, diabetes, and certain cardiac conditions (conduction problems) |
| Quetiapine | IR: 25–300 mg/d ER: 50–300 mg/d IR: 25–400 mg/d IR: 25–800 mg/d | Somnolence, dizziness, weight gain, and other long-term metabolic side effects | GAD OCD PTSD | **Antidepressants increase the risk of suicidal thinking and behavior in children, adolescents, and young adults (18–24 y of age) with MDD and other psychiatric disorders** |

*Abbreviations:* ER, extended release; IR, instant release; IV, intravenously; SNRI, serotonin-norepinephrine reuptake inhibitors; SSRI, selective serotonin reuptake inhibitors.

*Data from* Stahl SM. *Prescriber's Guide.* 6th ed. Cambridge, UK: Cambridge University Press; 2017 and Bystritsky A, Hermann R, Stein MB. Pharmacotherapy for generalized anxiety disorder. https://www.uptodate.com/contents/pharmacotherapy-for-generalized-anxiety-disorder-in-adults?search=pharmacology%20of%20anxiety%20disorders&source=search_result&selectedTitle=1~150&usage_type=default&display_rank=1. Updated August 31, 2018. Accessed December 18, 2018.

health and/or medical comorbidities, a high number of concomitant medications, or if there is concern for the patient's personal safety or safety of others. If safety concerns are imminent, emergent care should be obtained through the crisis center helpline or other available community resources. A validating, empathetic, and resourceful encounter is pertinent in helping to increase the likelihood of early intervention and treatment. Potential for improved treatment outcomes may be maximized by using evidence-based recommendations and guidelines in the pharmacologic approach. Selective serotonin reuptake inhibitors and serotonin-norepinephrine reuptake inhibitors are the preferred first-line treatments. Benzodiazepines should be used with caution and in short-term settings as adjuncts to initial pharmacologic treatment. All agents should be used after consideration of their risks and benefits to the patient in order to maximize patient compliance and treatment response.

## REFERENCES

1. Colorafi K, Vanselow J, Nelson T. Treating anxiety and depression in primary care: reducing barriers to access. Fam Pract Manag 2017;24(4):11–6. Available at: https://www.aafp.org/fpm/2017/0700/p11.pdf. Accessed November 18, 2018.
2. Kessler RC, Petukhova M, Sampson NA, et al. Twelve-month and lifetime prevalence and lifetime morbid risk of anxiety and mood disorders in the United States. Int J MethodsPsychiatr Res 2012;21(3):169–84.
3. Combs H, Markman J. Anxiety disorders in primary care. Med Clin North Am 2014;98(5):1007–23.
4. Shirneshan E, Bailey J, Relyea G, et al. Incremental direct medical expenditures associated with anxiety disorders for the U.S. adult population: evidence from the Medical Expenditure Panel Survey. J AnxietyDisord 2013;27(7):720–7.
5. Stein DJ, Lim CCW, Roest AM, et al, WHO World Mental Health Survey Collaborators. The cross-national epidemiology of social anxiety disorder: data from the World Mental Health Survey Initiative. BMC Med 2017;15(1):143.
6. Nutter DA, Jr. Pediatric generalized anxiety disorder medication. In: Pataki C, editor. Pediatrics: Developmental and Behavioral Articles. Medscape; 2017. Available at: https://emedicine.medscape.com/article/916933-overview#a3. Accessed November 5, 2018.
7. Sakolsky DJ, McCracken JT, Nurmi EL. Genetics of pediatric anxiety disorders. Child AdolescPsychiatrClin N Am 2012;21(3):479–500.
8. Bennett S, Walkup JT, Brent D, et al, editors. Anxiety disorders in children and adolescents: epidemiology, pathogenesis, clinical manifestations, and course. UpToDate; 2018. Available at: https://www.uptodate.com/contents/anxiety-disorders-in-children-and-adolescents-epidemiology-pathogenesis-clinical-manifestations-and-course. Accessed November 5, 2018.
9. Carlisi CO, Hilbert K, Guyer AE, et al. Sleep-amount differentially affects fear-processing neural circuitry in pediatric anxiety: a preliminary fMRI investigation. CognAffectBehavNeurosci 2017;17(6):1098–11113.
10. Klumpp H, Fitzgerald DA, Cook E, et al. Serotonin transporter gene alters insula activity to threat in social anxiety disorder. Neuroreport 2014;25(12):926–31.
11. Eley TC, McAdams TA, Rijsdijk FV, et al. The intergenerational transmission of anxiety: a children-of-twins study. Am J Psychiatry 2015;172(7):630–7.
12. Bekhuis E, Boschloo L, Rosmalen JG, et al. Differential associations of specific depressive and anxiety disorders with somatic symptoms. J Psychosom Res 2015;78(2):116–22.

13. Bandelow B, Sher L, Bunevicius R, et al, WFSBP Task Force on Mental Disorders in Primary Care, WFSBP Task Force on Anxiety Disorders, OCD and PTSD. Guidelines for the pharmacological treatment of anxiety disorders, obsessive-compulsive disorder and posttraumatic stress disorder in primary care. Int J PsychiatryClinPract 2012;16:77–84.

14. American Psychiatric Association. Diagnostic and statistical manual of mental disorders. 5th edition. Arlington (VA): American Psychiatric Association; 2013.

15. Baldwin D, Murray BS, Hermann R, editors. Generalized anxiety disorder in adults: epidemiology, pathogensis, clinical manifestations, course, assessment, and diagnosis. 2018. Available at: https://www.uptodate.com/contents/generalized-anxiety-disorder-in-adults-epidemiology-pathogenesis-clinical-manifestations-course-assessment-and-diagnosis. Accessed November 24, 2018.

16. Rivelli SK, Shirey KG. Prevalence of psychiatric symptoms/syndromes in medical settings. In: Summergrad P, Kathol RG, editors. Integrated care in psychiatry: redefining the role of mental health professionals in the medical setting. New York: Springer; 2014. p. 5–27.

17. Bandelow B, Michaelis S. Epidemiology of anxiety disorders in the 21st century. DialoguesClinNeurosci 2015;17(3):327–35.

18. Kwan E, Wijeratne C. Presentations of anxiety in older people. MedToday 2016; 17(12):34–41. Available at: https://medicinetoday.com.au/system/files/pdf/MT2016-12-034-KWAN.pdf. Accessed December 7, 2018.

19. Schneier FR, Stein MB, eds., Hermann R, eds.Social anxiety disorder in adults: epidemiology, clinical manifestations, and diagnosis. Available at: https://www.uptodate.com/contents/social-anxiety-disorder-in-adults-epidemiology-clinical-manifestations-and-diagnosis. 2017. Accessed November 24, 2018.

20. Bennett S, Walkup JT, Brent D, et al, editors. Anxiety disorders in children and adoelscents: assessment and diagnosis. 2018. Available at: https://www.uptodate.com/contents/anxiety-disorders-in-children-and-adolescents-epidemiology-pathogenesis-clinical-manifestations-and-course. Accessed December 15, 2018.

21. Lebens ML, Lauth GW. Risk and resilience factors of post-traumatic stress disorder: A review of current research. ClinExp Psychol 2016;2:120.

22. Alisic E, Zalta AK, van Wesel F, et al. Rates of post-traumatic stress disorder in trauma-exposed children and adolescents: meta-analysis. Br J Psychiatry 2014;204(5):335–40.

23. McLaughlin K, Brent D, Hermann R, editors. Posttraumatic stress disorder in children and adolescents: epidemiology, pathogenesis, clinical manifestations, course, assessment, and diagnosis. 2018. Available at: https://www.uptodate.com/contents/posttraumatic-stress-disorder-in-children-and-adolescents-epidemiology-pathogenesis-clinical-manifestations-course-assessment-and-diagnosis. Accessed November 20, 2018.

24. McLaughlin KA, Koenen KC, Hill ED, et al. Trauma exposure and posttraumatic stress disorder in a national sample of adolescents. J Am Acad Child Adolesc-Psychiatry 2013;52(8):815–30.e14.

25. Veale D, Roberts A. Obsessive compulsive disorder: a review. BMJ 2014;348:g2183.

26. Ruscio AM, Stein DJ, Chiu WT, et al. The epidemiology of obsessive-compulsive disorder in the National Comorbidity Survey Replication. MolPscyhiatry 2010; 15(1):53–63.

27. Rosenberg D, Brent D, Hermann R, editors. Obsessive-compulsive disorder in children and adolescents: epidemiology, pathogenesis, clinical manifestations, course, assessment, and diagnosis. 2017. Available at: http://wwwuptodate com.uptodate.qfsy.yuntsg.cn:7002/contents/obsessive-compulsive-disorder-in-

children-and-adolescents-epidemiology-pathogenesis-clinical-manifestations-course-assessment-and-diagnosis. Accessed December 10, 2018.

28. Singer HS, Gilbert DL, Wolf DS, et al. Moving from PANDAS to CANS. J Pediatr 2012;160(5):725–31.
29. Pan American Health Organization; World Health Organization. Health status of the population: mental health in the Americas. Available at: https://www.paho.org/salud-en-las-americas-2017/?p=1270. Accessed December 10, 2018.
30. Angelakis I, Gooding P, Tarrier N, et al. Suicidality in obsessive compulsive disorder (OCD): a systematic review and meta-analysis. ClinPsychol Rev 2015; 39:1–15.
31. National Institute of Mental Health. Anxiety disorders. Available at: https://www.nimh.nih.gov/health/topics/anxiety-disorders/index.shtml. Accessed November 3, 2018.
32. American Academy of Child and Adolescent Psychiatry. Panic disorder in children and adolescents. Available at: https://www.aacap.org/aacap/families_and_youth/facts_for_families/fff-guide/Panic-Disorder-In-Children-And-Adolescents-050.aspx. Accessed November 11, 2018.
33. Shirneshan E. Cost of illness study of anxiety disorders for the ambulatory adult population of the United States [dissertation]. University of Tennessee; 2013. p. 87. https://doi.org/10.21007/etd.cghs.2013.0289 [UTHSCdigital commons]. Paper 370.
34. Wahlin T, Deane F. Discrepancies between parent- and adolescent-perceived problem severity and influences on help seeking from mental health services. Aust N Z J Psychiatry 2012;46(6):553–60.
35. de Los Reyes A, Augenstein TM, Wang M, et al. The validity of the multi-informant approach to assessing child and adolescent mental health. Psychol Bull 2015; 141(4):858–900.
36. Beidas RS, Stewart RB, Walsh L, et al. Free, brief, and validated: Standardized instruments for low-resource mental health settings. CognBehavPract 2016; 22(1):5–19.
37. Jordan P, Shedden-Mora MC, Lowe B. Psychometric analysis of the Generalized Anxiety Disorder scale (GAD-7) in primary care using modern item response theory. PLoSOne 2017;12(8):e0182162.
38. Wuthrich VM, Johnco C, Knight A. Comparison of the Penn State Worry Questionnaire (PSWQ) and abbreviated version (PSWQ-A) in a clinical and non-clinical population of older adults. J AnxietyDisord 2014;28(7):657–63.
39. Arcangelo VP, Peterson AM, editors. Pharmacotherapeutics for advanced practice: a practical approach, vol. 536, 2ndedition. Philadelphia: Lippincott Williams & Wilkins; 2016.
40. Bandelow B, Lichte T, Rudolf S, et al. The German guidelines for the treatment of anxiety disorders. Eur Arch PsychiatryClinNeurosci 2015;265(5):363–73.
41. Mohatt J, Bennett SM, Walkup JT. Treatment of separation, generalized, and social anxiety disorders in youths. Am J Psychiatry 2014;171(1):741–8.
42. Wetherell JL, Petkus AJ, White KS, et al. Antidepressant medication augmented with cognitive-behavioral therapy for generalized anxiety disorder in older adults. Am J Psychiatry 2013;170(7):782–9.
43. Edwards MK, Rosenbaum S, Loprinzi PD. Differential experimental effects of a short bout of walking, meditation, or combination of walking and meditation on state anxiety among young adults. Am J HealthPromot 2018;32(4):949–58.
44. Stubbs B, Koyanagi A, Hallgren M, et al. Physical activity and anxiety: a perspective from the World Health Survey. J AffectDisord 2017;208:545–52.

45. Stubbs B, Vancampfort D, Rosenbaum S, et al. An examination of the anxiolytic effects of exercise for people with anxiety and stress-related disorders: a meta-analysis. Psychiatry Res 2017;249:102–8.
46. Bolognesi F, Baldwin DS, Ruini C. Psychological interventions in the treatment of generalized anxiety disorder: a structured review. J Psycho Pathol 2014;20:111–26.
47. Anderson E, Shivakumar G. Effects of exercise and physical activity on anxiety. Front Psychiatry 2013;4(27):1–4.
48. Mahmood L, Hopthrow T, Randsley de Moura G. A moment of mindfulness: computer-mediated mindfulness practice increases state mindfulness. PLoS One 2016;11(4):e0153923.
49. Johnson S, Gur RM, David Z, et al. One session mindfulness meditation: a randomized controlled study of effects on cognition and mood. Mindfulness 2015;6(1):88–98.

# A Brief Overview of Identification and Management of Opiate Use Disorder in the Primary Care Setting

Ian Thomas, DNP, PMHNP*

## KEYWORDS

- Opioid epidemic • Overdose • Opioid use disorder • Fentanyl • MAT
- Medication-assisted treatment

## KEY POINTS

- Opiate abuse presents significant challenges in the primary care setting, including a very high risk for mortality and morbidity.
- There are only 3 medications approved by the Food and Drug Administration for the treatment of opiate use disorder. Buprenorphine and methadone have significant regulatory barriers whereas naltrexone is available to most prescribers; however, referral to an addiction specialist is preferred.
- With the addition of illicitly produced fentanyl into common substances of abuse, lethality of overdose has increased while users and clinicians have no way of determining its presence
- Medication-assisted treatment is only part of a holistic treatment model, including talk therapy and likely inpatient and residential addiction treatment.

## INTRODUCTION

The purpose of this article is to summarize the most recent developments and recommendations for managing opiate use disorder, with an emphasis on the primary care setting. The goal is also to provide a summary of what treatment options are available and increase provider comfort when working with this challenging and vulnerable population. This article includes an outline of all 3 Food and Drug Administration–approved medications used in the treatment of opiate use disorder.[1] It also brings attention to

Disclosure: No disclosures.
Carondelet Health Network, 2656 North Sahuara Place, Tucson, AZ 85712, USA
* Corresponding author. 1601 W St Mary's Road, Tucson, AZ 85745.
E-mail address: IanThomas83@gmail.com

Nurs Clin N Am 54 (2019) 495–501
https://doi.org/10.1016/j.cnur.2019.08.006
0029-6465/19/© 2019 Elsevier Inc. All rights reserved.

both the scale of the current opiate epidemic and the potency of current substances of abuse in communities. Due to both the constantly increasing risk for fatal overdose and the high rate of psychiatric comorbidities in the population, it is important to recommend regular consultation with, and at times referral to, a psychiatric provider familiar with management of opiate use disorder or a certified addiction specialist. Furthermore, the best patient outcomes are achieved with an individualized and holistic approach that revolves around behavioral interventions and psychotherapy, preferably delivered by a psychologist or other licensed therapist familiar with treating addictions. Use of medication-assisted treatment (MAT) with methadone, buprenorphine, and naltrexone are best used as methods of harm reduction and to keep patients engaged in treatment and are considered adjuncts to intensive talk therapy delivered both individually and in group settings as well as in residential, intensive outpatient, and partial hospitalization programs.

It is difficult to overstate the magnitude of the current opioid epidemic in the United States. Currently, Americans are more likely to die from an opiate overdose than they are from a motor vehicle collision.[2] From 2001 to 2016, total opioid-related deaths increased by approximately 350%.[3] In 2017 alone, approximately 72,000 people died from any drug overdose and more than 29,000 of those were from synthetic opioids, predominantly fentanyl.[4] These trends continue to worsen every year while opioids and other synthetic drugs of abuse grow in potency and availability.

## CLINICAL ASSESSMENT

Accurate screening for illicit substance abuse in the primary care setting has been a challenge and historically more difficult than screening for alcohol and tobacco. This is likely related to the legal status and social stigma associated with substances of abuse. For many patients, disclosing the illicit use of substances of abuse to a health care provider can feel as though they are admitting to a crime. Current recommendations suggest that screening, brief intervention, and referral to treatment (SBIRT) be used to identify and treat patients with substance use disorders in the primary care setting. Essentially, the goal of using SBIRT is to positively identify patients who are at risk of a substance use disorders and then stratify the level of risk into categories low, moderate, and high. Patients identified as low risk can be provided brief intervention in the form of education, highlighting the dangers and health risks of substance abuse. Moderate-risk and high-risk patients should be given the same education in the form of brief intervention but also receive a referral to specialized addictions treatment.

The single-question screening tool is both fast and effective in the primary care setting.[5] Asking "How many times in the past year have you used an illegal drug or used a prescription medication for nonmedical reasons?" serves to separate patients who are at risk of a substance use disorder and those who are not. Any answer indicating 1 or more times in a year is a positive screen for substance abuse risk. If positive, the clinician moves onto the recommended and free tool published by the National Institute on Drug Abuse (NIDA), the NIDA-Modified ASSIST questionnaire (**Fig. 1**). This tool then assesses lifetime drug use by category and identifies the level of risk. There is also a free online version of the NIDA-Modified ASSIST available at https://www.drugabuse.gov/nmassist/. The single-question screening tool assesses the misuse of drugs within the past year whereas the NIDA-Modified ASSIST assesses lifetime patterns of misuse. The risk level then directs the clinician to the appropriate response. Patients at low risk can be provided education and continuing support and benefit from reinforcing abstinence. Moderate-risk patients receive all the low-risk

| Question 1 of 8, NIDA-Modified ASSIST | Yes | No |
|---|---|---|
| **In your _LIFETIME_, which of the following substances have you ever used?**<br>*Note for Physicians: For prescription medications, please report nonmedical use only.* | | |
| a. **Cannabis** (marijuana, pot, grass, hash, etc.) | | |
| b. **Cocaine** (coke, crack, etc.) | | |
| c. **Prescription stimulants** (Ritalin, Concerta, Dexedrine, Adderall, diet pills, etc.) | | |
| d. **Methamphetamine** (speed, crystal meth, ice, etc.) | | |
| e. **Inhalants** (nitrous oxide, glue, gas, paint thinner, etc.) | | |
| f. **Sedatives or sleeping pills** (Valium, Serepax, Ativan, Xanax, Librium,Rohypnol, GHB, etc.) | | |
| g. **Hallucinogens** (LSD, acid, mushrooms, PCP, Special K, ecstasy, etc.) | | |
| h. **Street opioids** (heroin, opium, etc.) | | |
| i. **Prescription opioids** (fentanyl, oxycodone [OxyContin, Percocet], hydrocodone [Vicodin], methadone, buprenorphine, etc.) | | |
| j. **Other – specify:** | | |

**Fig. 1.** First of 8 questions used in the NIDA-Modified ASSIST risk assessment tool. (*Courtesy of* National Institute on Drug Abuse. Available at: https://www.drugabuse.gov/sites/default/files/pdf/nmassist.pdf.)

interventions, and clinicians also should consider referral to an addiction specialist. The high-risk category patients receive the same interventions, with the exception that specialist referral is not optional and should be made as soon as possible, preferably before the patient leaves the clinic that day.

## MEDICATION-ASSISTED TREATMENT

At this time, there are 3 medications approved for the treatment of opiate use disorder: buprenorphine, methadone, and naltrexone.[1] Each of these drugs represents 1 of 3 distinct mechanisms of action at the opioid receptor: full agonist, agonist/antagonist, and full antagonist; they are described later. All 3 treatment modalities show similar efficacy in terms of treatment and abstinence compared with placebo. The advantages of MAT are reduced mortality, reduced risk of overdose, reduced exposure to human immunodeficiency virus, and decreased relapse compared with treatment without medication.

Prescribing the opiate agonist methadone and the agonist/antagonist buprenorphine requires extensive extra licensing, and they typically are available only through substance abuse specialty providers. The opiate antagonist naltrexone, however, is available to all prescribers. Finally, although not considered a MAT, naloxone also is a critical harm reduction component of treating patients suffering from opiate use disorder and is described as well.

- Methadone is a full opioid agonist and the oldest approved medication for the management of opiate abuse disorder. It is associated with increased number of days in treatment and decreased incidence of relapse. In rare circumstances, this medication can be used to manage chronic pain in cancer and noncancer patients. Methadone is highly regulated, which creates significant barriers for the facility, provider, and patients. Specifically, methadone is required to be dosed out from a specialized methadone clinic that must overcome significant regulatory requirements; providers must obtain certification; and patients usually are required to travel to the clinics every 24 hours to receive their prescribed dose. This regimen makes it difficult for patients to have flexibility for travel, employment, and in their general lives.

- Buprenorphine—this medication is an opiate agonist/antagonist and is considered safer than methadone in terms of all-cause mortality and acute poisoning.[6] Also, overdose is considered more difficult and less lethal because, unlike methadone, buprenorphine is thought to be limited in its ability to cause respiratory depression. The safety benefits of buprenorphine, however, are not as straightforward as once believed and data from France where buprenorphine is used more commonly and at greater doses have shown that fatal overdose with buprenorphine not only is possible but also seems more common than expected.[7] One complicating factor is that buprenorphine overdose is not as responsive to naloxone and, although overdose is not as lethal compared with methadone directly, some evidence suggests buprenorphine overdoses are more lethal compared with methadone if used in combinations with sedatives like benzodiazepines.[7] Prescription privileges of buprenorphine are granted only through special license from the Drug Enforcement Administration but it has significantly fewer regulatory barriers than methadone.

- Naltrexone—naltrexone is a long-acting full opioid antagonist and can decrease the desire and craving for opiates.[8,9] It is contraindicated before detoxification is completed and should not be prescribed until a patient has not used opioids for at least 7 days. Primarily, it is available both orally and by intramuscular injection. Naltrexone can be taken orally once a day (50 mg) or once every other day (100 mg). Naltrexone is delivered through intramuscular injection dosed approximately every 4 weeks. In the United States the average cost of the injection can be prohibitive for some at $1309/months[8] while in the United States 30 tablets cost approximately $60. Other contraindications for naltrexone are patients with liver failure and patients whose pain management requires opiate medications. Fatal opiate overdose while on naltrexone is possible in a patient who takes excessive amounts of opioids such that they overcome the antagonist blockade. There also is evidence that after taking naltrexone, opiate tolerance is quickly and dramatically decreased, leading to a rebound risk of overdose, especially if patients return to their previous doses of opiates.[10]

- Naloxone—this medication is a short-acting full opioid antagonist and is not considered to be MAT. It is used during emergencies to reverse the fatal effects of opiate overdose, primarily respiratory depression, thereby preventing mortality. It is the only medication used to reverse opiate overdose and is on the World Health Organization list of essential medicines.[11] More recently, it has been recommended that naloxone prescriptions be provided to both patients and their loved ones in order to have easy and quick access to the lifesaving medication should patients experience an overdose.[12,13] When given intravenously or intramuscularly, the onset is between 2 minutes and 5 minutes and can last up to 1 hour. More potent drugs like fentanyl and fentanyl analogs may require several naloxone doses to adequately reverse overdose.[14] Also, vials of the generic medication cost less than $20 but new autoinjectors and nasal sprays can cost up to $4500 a dose.

## DRUGS OF ABUSE

The Substance Abuse and Mental Health Services Administration has indicated that the number of new heroin users was down to approximately 81,000 new users in 2017; however, first-time misuse of prescription opioid medications has remained relatively stable since 2015, at 2 million new users a year.[15] There may be some encouragement in these numbers from a public health standpoint, but these numbers also demonstrate the enormity of the opioid abuse problem. Although heroin abuse seems to be trending down on a global scale, since the early 2000s, heroin has been making new appearances in demographics not usually associated with opiate abuse, namely women and high-income households.[16] Also concerning is that frequently when patients believe they are buying heroin or diverted pharmaceutical-grade medication on the street, they are unknowingly buying illicitly produced fentanyl or a fentanyl analog.[17] In addition to the high mortality and morbidity of fentanyl abuse, there is no widely available Food and Drug Administration–approved test for fentanyl metabolites. Therefore, clinically speaking, patients may be regularly abusing fentanyl when presenting with or without a chief complaint related to opiate abuse and test negative on urine toxicology.

Fentanyl/fentanyl analogs—fentanyl has become its own epidemic within an epidemic.[18] Fentanyl is problematic on several levels:

It is cheap and easy to create illicitly.

Due to its high potency, it can be easily transported in bulk using smaller-volume containers relative to other drugs like heroin.

It is easily added to other drugs of abuse and is misrepresented as pharmaceutical medication, such as prescription opiates and alprazolam.[19,20]

Fatal heroin overdose can occur within 30 minutes after injection whereas fentanyl may take only 2 minutes.[13]

Fentanyl overdose is resistant to naloxone reversal and requires higher and more frequent doses.[13]

Fentanyl is up to 40 times more powerful than heroin, and fentanyl analogs can be 4000 times stronger.[21]

Given the high potency of fentanyl and fentanyl analogs, the lethal dose is quite low relative to heroin (**Fig. 2**).

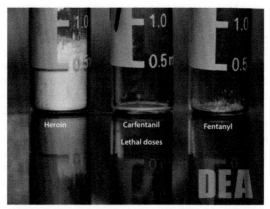

**Fig. 2.** Visual comparison of lethal doses (*left* to *right*) of heroin, carfentanil and fentanyl. (*Courtesy of* United States Drug Enforcement Administration. Available at: https://www.dea.gov/galleries/drug-images/fentanyl.)

Fentanyl is uniquely problematic because patients may not be aware they are taking it. Instead, they may believe they are using pharmaceutical-grade alprazolam or oxycodone.[17,18,21] Cocaine and methamphetamine frequently are adulterated with fentanyl as well. The Drug Enforcement Administration has reported deaths by fentanyl more than tripled between 2014 and 2015 and the trend continues to rise. Heroin abuse and fentanyl abuse are becoming interlinked, possibly inseparable; combined with the fact that 75% of new heroin users abused prescription opioid medication before using heroin and that prescription opioids are becoming more tightly regulated, it appears that more patients are turning to heroin when prescription opioids are not available.[21]

## SUMMARY

To summarize, the opiate epidemic continues to grow and evolve in the United States. Few treatment options exist, and patients require robust treatment plans delivered by multidisciplinary professional teams and, for more severe cases, residential treatment with MAT using methadone, buprenorphine, or naltrexone. Although access to methadone and buprenorphine can be challenging, access to naltrexone and naloxone is essentially wide open. Fentanyl has brought new challenges to the world of opiate use disorder, and its high lethality, high potency, and nearly ubiquitous presence in both opiate and nonopiate drugs of abuse make detection and recognition difficult and sometimes impossible. Patients at risk of or suspected to be struggling with opiate use disorder should be rapidly identified and referred to specialized treatment using SBIRT and, when appropriate, prescribed the overdose reversal medication naloxone.

## REFERENCES

1. U.S. Food and Drug Administration. Information about Medication-Assisted Treatment (MAT) 2018. Available at: https://www.fda.gov/Drugs/DrugSafety/InformationbyDrugClass/ucm600092.htm.
2. National Safety Council. For the first time, we're more likely to die from accidental opioid overdose than motor vehicle crash 2019. Available at: https://www.prnewswire.com/news-releases/for-the-first-time-were-more-likely-to-die-from-accidental-opioid-overdose-than-motor-vehicle-crash-300777184.html.
3. Gomes T, Tadrous M, Mamdani MM, et al. The burden of opioid-related mortality in the united statesthe burden of opioid-related mortality in the United States, 2001-2016 the burden of opioid-related mortality in the United States, 2001-2016. JAMA Netw Open 2018;1(2):e180217.
4. National Institute on Drug Abuse. Overdose death rates 2018. Available at: https://www.drugabuse.gov/related-topics/trends-statistics/overdose-death-rates.
5. Smith PC, Schmidt SM, Allensworth-Davies D, et al. A single-question screening test for drug use in primary care. Arch Intern Med 2010;170(13):1155–60.
6. Hickman M, Steer C, Tilling K, et al. The impact of buprenorphine and methadone on mortality: a primary care cohort study in the United Kingdom. Addiction 2018; 113(8):1461–76.
7. Sansone RA, Sansone LA. Buprenorphine treatment for narcotic addiction: not without risks. Innov Clin Neurosci 2015;12(3–4):32–6.
8. Ndegwa S, Pant S, Pohar S, et al. Injectable extended-release naltrexone to treat opioid use disorder. In: CADTH issues in emerging health technologies. Ottawa (ON): Canadian Agency for Drugs and Technologies in Health; 2016. p. 1–14. Available at. https://www.ncbi.nlm.nih.gov/pubmed/29400929.

9. Bigelow GE, Preston KL, Schmittner J, et al. Opioid challenge evaluation of blockade by extended-release naltrexone in opioid-abusing adults: dose-effects and time-course. Drug Alcohol Depend 2012;123(1–3):57–65.
10. Saucier R, Wolfe D, Dasgupta N. Review of case narratives from fatal overdoses associated with injectable naltrexone for opioid dependence. Drug Saf 2018; 41(10):981–8.
11. World Health Organization. The WHO model lists of essential medicines 2017. Available at: https://www.who.int/medicines/publications/essentialmedicines/ EML_2015_FINAL_amended_NOV2015.pdf?ua=1.
12. Adams JM. Increasing naloxone awareness and use: the role of health care practitioners. JAMA 2018;319(20):2073–4.
13. Fairbairn N, Coffin PO, Walley AY. Naloxone for heroin, prescription opioid, and illicitly made fentanyl overdoses: challenges and innovations responding to a dynamic epidemic. Int J Drug Policy 2017;46:172–9.
14. Somerville NJ, O'Donnell J, Gladden RM, et al. Characteristics of Fentanyl Overdose - Massachusetts, 2014-2016. MMWR Morb Mortal Wkly Rep 2017;66(14): 382–6.
15. Bose J, Hedden S, Lipari R, et al. Key substance use and mental health indicators in the United States: results from the 2017 national survey on drug use and health. Rockville (MD): Center for Behavioral Health Statistics and Quality, Substance Abuse and Mental Health Services Administration: Substance Abuse and Mental Health Services Administration; 2018.
16. Jones CM, Logan J, Gladden RM, et al. Vital signs: demographic and substance use trends among heroin users—United States, 2002–2013. MMWR Morbidity and mortality weekly report 2015;64(26):719.
17. O'Donnell J, Gladden R, Seth P. Trends in deaths involving heroin and synthetic opioids excluding methadone, and law enforcement drug product reports, by census region — United States, 2006–2015. U.S. Department of Health and Human Services; 2017.
18. Kuczynska K, Grzonkowski P, Kacprzak L, et al. Abuse of fentanyl: an emerging problem to face. Forensic Sci Int 2018;289:207–14.
19. Green TC, Gilbert M. Counterfeit medications and fentanyl. JAMA Intern Med 2016;176(10):1555–7.
20. Pichini S, Solimini R, Berretta P, et al. Acute intoxications and fatalities from illicit fentanyl and analogues: an update. Ther Drug Monit 2018;40(1):38–51.
21. O'Donnell J, Gladden RM, Mattson CL, et al. Notes from the field: overdose deaths with carfentanil and other fentanyl analogs detected — 10 states, July 2016–June 2017. MMWR Morb Mortal Wkly Rep 2018;67(27):767–8.

# Military Service–Related Post-traumatic Stress Disorder: Finding a Way Home

Pamela Herbig Wall, PhD, PMHNP-BC[a],
Sean P. Convoy, DNP, PMHNP-BC[b,1],
Connie J. Braybrook, DNP, PMHNP-BC[c],*

## KEYWORDS

- Post-traumatic stress disorder • Military service members • Trauma informed care

## KEY POINTS

- Disease states related to traumatic experiences can be a cause of disability and morbidity.
- Pathophysiological concepts, trauma informed care, and evidence-based treatments are discussed as a path to recovery.
- Today, veterans are exposed to a multitude of operational, occupational, and interpersonal stresses that negatively affect far too many aspects of their health and well-being.

## INTRODUCTION

Military service, war, and the struggle to find one's way home has been chronicled in literature since before the time of Homer (**Box 1**).[1] Although the literature has done an exemplary job of describing the phenomenon of stress born of military service and war, less has been done to understand, treat, and prevent its sequelae. Today,

Disclosure Statement: The views expressed in this article reflect the results of research conducted by the authors and do not necessarily reflect the official policy or position of the Department of the Navy, Department of Defense, or the United States Government. Neither the Department of the Navy nor any other component of the Department of Defense has approved, endorsed, or authorized this article.

This article is dedicated to our fellow Naval Officer Veterans' President (Lieutenant) H.W. Bush and Senator (Captain, ret) John McCain. Thank you for your service, CAVU (ceiling and visibility unlimited), you can rest now, we have the watch. CDR (ret) Sean P. Convoy, CDR (ret) Pam Wall, and CDR Connie Braybrook.

[a] United States Government, 8600 Harrington Place, Sanford, NC 27332, USA; [b] Duke School of Nursing, DUMC 3322, Room 2015, 307 Trent Drive, Durham, NC 27710, USA; [c] United States Navy, Naval Branch Health Clinic Fallon, 4755 Pasture Road, Building 299, Fallon, NV 89496, USA

[1] Present address: 2900 Mills Lake Wynd, Holly Springs, NC 27540.

* Corresponding author. DUMC 3322, Room 2015, 307 Trent Drive, Durham, NC 27710.

E-mail address: connie.j.braybrook.mil@mail.mil

---

**Box 1**
**Homer, the Odyssey**

Sing to me of the man, Muse, the man of twists and turns ... driven time and again off course, once he had plundered the hallowed heights of Troy. Many cities of men he saw and learned their minds, many pains he suffered, heartsick on the open sea, fighting to save his life and bring his comrades home.

*From* Griffin J. Homer: The Odyssey. Cambridge, UK: Cambridge University Press; 2004; with permission.

---

veterans are exposed to a multitude of operational, occupational, and interpersonal stresses that negatively affect far too many aspects of their health and well-being. Mental illness and injury, including post-traumatic stress disorder (PTSD), represents a significant source of disability and morbidity among military and veteran populations. Mental illness and injury have been a primary cause of medical evacuations and in-theater hospitalizations among our generation's recent war campaigns.[2,3] Mental illness and injury was responsible for 40.1% of all military hospital bed days and ranked as the third or fourth most common reason for military ambulatory visits in the years 2007, 2009, and 2011.[4] The suicide rate among the veteran population disproportionately contributes to the nation's suicide rate with approximately 20 completed suicides per day. Among active duty and reserve/national guard, the suicide rate for CY2016 was 21.1 and 22.0 per 100,000, respectively.[5] Combined, the behavioral health needs of the active, reserve, and guard components and their veteran brethren are staggering. The evidence suggests that rural veterans appear to be particularly vulnerable because they are less likely to use behavioral health services because of structural barriers to care. Overall in the United States veterans constitute 10.4% of the adult rural population as compared with 7.8% of the adult urban population.[6] The veteran population's unique culture and background, by definition, make it a vulnerable population.

## POST-TRAUMATIC STRESS DISORDER
### Epidemiology of Post-traumatic Stress Disorder

Exposure to a traumatic event is significant; national estimates of traumatic event exposure in the United States is 89.7%,[7] with men more likely to be exposed to trauma than women (26%–81% versus 17%–74%).[7–9] The prevalence of PTSD among Vietnam veterans rages from 2% to 17%.[10,11] Prevalence rates for PTSD among those who served during contemporary wars (**Table 1**) range between 4% and 17%.[12,13]

---

**Table 1**
**American veteran-supported contemporary wars**

| Military Campaign | Years | Geographic Location |
|---|---|---|
| Iraqi no-fly zone enforcement operations | 1991–2003 | Persian Gulf |
| Operation Enduring Freedom (OEF) | 2001–2014 | Afghanistan, Philippines, Horn of Africa, & Guantanamo Bay, Cuba |
| Operational Iraqi Freedom (OIF) | 2003–2010 | Kuwait, Iraq |
| Operation New Dawn (OND) | 2010–2011 | Kuwait, Iraq |
| Operation Inherent Resolve (OIR) | 2014–Present | Iraq, Syria |

The increased incidence and prevalence of PTSD among OIF (Operation Iraqi Freedom) and OEF (Operation Enduring Freedom) veterans is not yet sufficiently understood but likely multifactorial in nature. Risk factors associated with PTSD among veteran populations include being female, of younger age, of enlisted rank, not being in a relationship, of low education, with history of childhood adversity, with low social support, being deployed more than once, being deployed to a forward area, higher combat exposure, being injured, being in the national guard or reserve, and being in the Army or Navy.[14–17]

PTSD is a neuropsychiatric condition nested within the *Diagnostic and Statistical Manual of Mental Disorders*, 5th Edition (DSM5)[18] Trauma and Stressor-Related Disorder classification. Informed by clinical observation of individuals exposed to natural and man-made disasters, current DSM5 criteria for PTSD require exposure to clinically significant trauma with resultant symptoms of intrusion, avoidance, and alternations in cognition, mood, arousal, and reactivity. General population lifetime prevalence is 3.5% to 7.8%[8,19] with a past year incidence of 3.5%.[20] Although men report more frequent exposure to traumatic events, women seem to be more likely to suffer from the disorder.[8,21] Other risk factors for the development of PTSD include socioeconomic status, education, intelligence level, race (eg, Hispanic, African American, American Indian, and Pacific Islander), childhood trauma, previous traumatization, adverse childhood events, familial mental illness, physical injury during the inferred index trauma, and lack of social support.[22]

### Pathophysiologic Impact of Post-traumatic Stress Disorder

Although science has not yet definitively explained why some are more vulnerable to PTSD than others, there is general consensus revolving around the epigenetic relationship that includes genomic vulnerability, adverse childhood events, established mental illness, and trauma exposure. The pathophysiologic mechanism of action of PTSD is associated with dysfunction(s) within the hypothalamic-pituitary-adrenal (HPA) axis, deficits in arousal and sleep-regulating systems, and problems within the endogenous opioid system of the brain.[23] PTSD can manifest in response to intense and/or protracted stress as defined by DSM5, criterion A. It is in response to this trauma (criterion A) that pathophysiologic changes in the brain dysregulate the HPA axis, which leads to symptoms of intrusion (criterion B) and alterations in arousal and reactivity (criterion E). Through the post-traumatic recapitulation of the inferred index trauma(s), negative alterations in cognition and mood (criterion D) and avoidance (criterion C) manifest. In essence, PTSD starts as an acute neurochemical stress attack on the brain that can, given the wrong circumstances, chronically persist through learning, reinforcement, and persisting HPA axis dysregulation subsequent to post-traumatic triggering. PTSD can manifest acutely, chronically, with delayed expression, and subclinically. Its symptom expression can tidal above and below the clinical threshold indefinitely in response to relative degrees of biopsychosocial stability. Evidence suggests that the greater the negative epigenetic weight, the more likely the condition will manifest chronically with increased symptom and functional burden. Although longitudinal studies are sparse, those groups that have been studied show disease course fluctuation[24] and increased chronicity with co-occurring mental health disorders,[25,26] and those with chronic PTSD have worse mental health quality-of-life indicators.[26]

PTSD includes 2 sleep disturbances as part of its diagnostic criteria. There is conflicting evidence as to whether sleep disturbances are a precursor of PTSD[27]; however, sleep disturbances around the time of the traumatic incident have been shown to predict future symptomatology. Seventy percent to 87% of those diagnosed with

PTSD experience sleep disturbances,[28,29] mostly in the form of nightmares or problems falling or staying asleep. Not only are sleep disturbances early predictors of PTSD[30] but they also greatly contribute to symptom severity and perceived mental health.[24]

## INTERVENTIONS FOR POST-TRAUMATIC STRESS DISORDER
### Trauma Informed Care

Clinically significant trauma exposure influences how an individual perceives self, others, and the world around them. The trauma symptom constructs of intrusion (criterion B), avoidance (criterion C), negative alterations in cognition and mood (criterion D), and alteration in arousal and reactivity (criterion E) are particularly relevant because they relates to fostering and maintaining therapeutic relationships with those exposed to trauma. Most patient-provider relationships are defined by unnatural degrees of one-sided physical and psychological intimacy, exposure, and vulnerability, given that the very nature of the therapeutic relationship can serve as a triggering event and unwittingly foster the disintegration of the therapeutic alliance.[31–33] To alleviate this, trauma informed care (TIC) is offered as an organizational structure and treatment framework that involves understanding, recognizing, and responding to the effects of trauma, however defined.[32] TIC is best conceptualized as a universal approach (or standard precaution) to delivering care. Substance Abuse and Mental Health Services Administration offers a scalable TIC framework with a set of principles, approaches, and interventions relevant to the discussion (**Table 2**).[31] Principles serve as cognitive and behavioral lodestars for clinical practice. Approaches aspire to raise awareness of trauma and its sequelae in the delivery of health care. Lastly, interventions codify specific behaviors that are internally consistent with TIC. The viability and sustainability of TIC depends on the adopting organizations' values and beliefs, leadership, community partnerships, and ongoing monitoring and evaluation of the interventions and programs for opportunities and successes.[31]

Using TIC with veterans potentially represents one aspect of "sea-change" (see https://www.youtube.com/watch?v=GsCnLX0LEko).

## TRANSITION FROM ASSESSMENT TO TREATMENT
### Diagnosing and Treating Across the Trajectory of Care

It is critical to both assess and understand where the patient is in relation to his or her trauma before setting out to treat it. Variables associated with chronology, co-occurrence, and comorbidity suggest that a plan of care uncommonly falls cleanly into a proprietary clinical practice guideline (CPG). Differentiation between acute, chronic, and delayed expressions of trauma has a real-time impact on clinical decision making. Timing of treatment is likely as important as the treatment itself. Many of the aforementioned evidence-based psychotherapies will only generate a clinically significant response if sequenced thoughtfully and executed effectively. Mindful of the pathophysiology, earnest attempts to use trauma-focused psychotherapy too soon represents a fool's errand. In the event of an acute presentation, the evidence suggests a period of decompression with focus on self-care, stress reduction, social connectedness, and (if indicated) crude target symptom stabilization with psychotropic medication before the initiation of trauma-focused therapy. Alternatively, chronic and delayed expressions of PTSD incline the provider to assess those compensatory, and commonly dysfunctional, behaviors the patient has been using to cope with trauma symptoms before engaging trauma-focused therapy as well. A commonly

**Table 2**
**Trauma informed care (TIC) principles, approach, and interventions**

| Principles | Clinical Application |
|---|---|
| 1. Safety<br>2. Trustworthiness & transparency<br>3. Peer support<br>4. Collaboration & mutuality<br>5. Empowerment, Voice & choice<br>6. Cultural, historical, and gender issues | 1. Considering TIC with environment of care decisions in the health care setting<br>2. Establishing limits of privacy and confidentiality with all patients prior to assessment<br>3. Recommending, coordinating, and praising the use of peer support systems to augment care delivery<br>4. Embracing principles of concordance with the patient and family when it comes to medical decision making<br>5. Soliciting and praising assertive behavior and evidence of self-efficacy in recovery<br>6. Resisting implicit bias associated with the delivery of care |

| Approach | Clinical Application |
|---|---|
| 1. *Realizes* the widespread impact of trauma and understands potential paths for recovery.<br>2. *Recognizes* the signs and symptoms of trauma in clients, families, staff, and others involved with the system<br>3. *Responds* by fully integrating knowledge about trauma into policies, procedures, and practices<br>4. Seeks to actively *resist re-traumatization* | 1. Considers, explores and anticipates the secondary and tertiary order consequences of trauma exposure and its sequelae intent to delimit the same.<br>2. Considers the varied expressions of trauma(s) and how it can manifest differently across the lifespan.<br>3. Translates TIC into all aspects of care from the waiting room to the examination room to social media.<br>4. Solicits feedback from patients and employs provider based after action reviews to critically analyze opportunities to improve TIC informed clinical practice. |

| Intervention | Clinical Application |
|---|---|
| Trauma-specific intervention programs generally recognize the following:<br>1. The survivor's need to be respected, informed, connected, and hopeful regarding their own recovery<br>2. The interrelation between trauma and symptoms of trauma such as substance abuse, eating disorders, depression, and anxiety<br>3. The need to work in a collaborative way with survivors, family and friends of the survivor, and other human services agencies in a manner that will empower survivors and consumers | 1. Explicitly recognize and acknowledge the trauma with unconditional positive regard and verbal, nonverbal, and paraverbal congruence<br>2. Anticipate and assess for high-volume and problem-prone comorbid and co-occurring illness associated with trauma- and stressor-related disorder<br>3. Translate clinical impact outside of the clinical space through TIC advocacy at the organizational, regional, and national level. Champion success stories that destigmatize and foster a sense of hope and universality |

used aphorism in clinical practice is to "never take away a defense mechanism you can't otherwise replace."

Gratefully, the evidence associated with the treatment of trauma-related and stressor-related disorders is now sufficiently robust to yield evidence-based CPGs. CPGs provide necessary structure to implement treatment, particularly for those who are new to the profession or are inexperienced in treating a particular condition. As previously established, CPGs in psychiatry should not be seen as a binary decision-making algorithm but rather a framework from which to practice. The Department of Defense (DoD) and Veterans Affairs (VA) provide some of the most comprehensive CPGs for the management of PTSD.

The VA/DoD CPGs gathered all research available through March 2016 to develop best practices to treat the symptoms of PTSD.[34] Grading of evidence was developed to indicate strong, weak, or no recommendation with regard to the workgroup, recommending a particular option for treatment. **Table 3** is a table from the CPG with the workgroup's recommendation regarding strength of evidence for treatment demonstrating consistency among studies (cognitive processing therapy, prolonged exposure, eye movement desensitization and reprocessing, brief eclectic psychotherapy,

| Table 3 Treatment of PTSD strength | | |
|---|---|---|
| **DoD/VA Clinical Practice Guideline Recommendations for the Treatment of PTSD** | | |
| **Recommendation** | | **Strength** |
| 1. | We recommend individual, manualized trauma-focused psychotherapy over other pharmacologic and non pharmacologic interventions for the primary treatment of PTSD | Strong for |
| 2. | When individual trauma-focused psychotherapy is not readily available or not preferred, we recommend pharmacotherapy or individual nontrauma-focused psychotherapy. With respect to pharmacotherapy and nontrauma-focused psychotherapy, there is insufficient evidence to recommend one over the other | Strong for |
| 3. | For patients with PTSD, we recommend individual, manualized trauma-focused psychotherapies that have a primary component of exposure and/or cognitive restructuring to include Prolonged Exposure (PE), Cognitive Processing Therapy (CPT), Eye Movement Desensitization and Reprocessing (EMDR), specific cognitive behavioral therapies for PTSD, Brief Eclectic Psychotherapy (BEP), Narrative Exposure Therapy (NET), and written narrative exposure | Strong for |
| 4. | We suggest the following individual, manualized nontrauma-focused therapies for patients diagnosed with PTSD: Stress Inoculation Training (SIT), Present-Centered Therapy (PCT), and Interpersonal Psychotherapy (IPT) | Weak for |
| 5. | There is insufficient evidence to recommend for or against psychotherapies that are not specified in other recommendations, such as Dialectical Behavior Therapy (DBT), Skills Training in Affect and Interpersonal Regulation (STAIR), Acceptance and Commitment Therapy (ACT), Seeking Safety, and supportive counseling | N/A |
| 6. | There is insufficient evidence to recommend using individual components of manualized psychotherapy protocols over or in addition to the full therapy protocol | N/A |
| 7. | We suggest manualized group therapy over no treatment. There is insufficient evidence to recommend using one type of group therapy over any other | Weak for |
| 8. | There is insufficient evidence to recommend for or against trauma-focused or nontrauma-focused couples therapy for the primary treatment of PTSD | N/A |

*Adapted from* The Management of Posttraumatic Stress Disorder Work Group. VA/DoD clinical practice guideline for the management of posttraumatic stress disorder and acute stress disorder. Department of Veterans Affairs. Department of Defense. Version 3.0. 2017; 33–34. Available at: https://www.healthquality.va.gov/guidelines/MH/ptsd/VADoDPTSDCPGFinal.pdf.

narrative exposure therapy), which have been the most studied and considered based on evidence (**Table 3**).

## Trauma informed psychotherapy

Evidenced-based treatment for PTSD includes cognitive behavioral therapy (CBT), cognitive processing therapy (CPT), prolonged exposure (PE), and adaptive disclosure therapy (ADT). These trauma informed therapies focus on either the memory of the traumatic event and/or its meaning by using different cognitive and behavioral techniques to help individuals process their trauma experience and its relative meaning. CBT, CPT, and PE currently have more robust evidence supporting their efficacy in comparison with others. Among the 49% to 70% who receive a full course of CPT and PE, clinical improvement has been reported.[35] Barriers to successful psychotherapeutic treatment include lengthy treatment protocols and high dropout rates.[36–38] A summary of each trauma informed psychotherapeutic treatment is presented in **Table 4**.

## Trauma informed pharmacotherapy

It may be helpful to conceptualize the brain as a master pharmacist of sorts. More often than not, the brain usually finds a way to self-regulate endogenously. In those instances where health care providers have to assist the master pharmacist, one's guidance is to never forget who is in charge and only do enough to help the master pharmacist re-engage. It is important to remember that psychotropic medications essentially alter how DNA is transcribed into messenger RNA. This realization should give pause to capricious prescribing. That being said, the use of psychotropic medications for this patient population is reasonably well established by the evidence. However, a clinician will likely obtain a better clinical response by focusing on symptom constitution over diagnostic label. PTSD criteria B through E constitute the phenotype of a trauma- and stressor-related disorder. The degree of symptomatic intensity, duration, and functional impairment associated with each criterion can vary greatly. In this regard, each trauma case is as unique as a fingerprint. Making general psychotropic decisions by diagnostic label makes about as much sense as prescribing an antibiotic for a case of sepsis without the benefit of a set of blood cultures. Clinicians are encouraged to deconstruct the presenting trauma symptoms and associate them with their corresponding brain region, neural circuit, and neurotransmitters. Once the presenting symptoms have been deconstructed down to their pathophysiologic point of origin, the clinician needs only to use those psychotropic medications that are known to effectively target the symptom construct as it presents. **Table 5** reflects a list psychotropic medications that are indicated for the symptomatic treatment of trauma-related and stressor-related disorders.

It is the authors' explicit intention to offer a short but effective list of psychotropic medications that predominately subsists within Food and Drug Administration (FDA) guidelines. Although the use of antipsychotic, mood stabilizer, and sedative-hypnotic agents unfortunately remain commonplace in clinical practice, they are not recommended. If they are to be used, it should be in the context of treating those symptoms that exist within co-occurring psychiatric condition sets (eg, PTSD and Bipolar, Schizophrenia Spectrum, or Depressive Disorders). More declaratively, the longitudinal use of benzodiazepine agents is now contraindicated because of their risk for dementia.[43,45]

How to approach the pharmacologic treatment of trauma-spectrum symptoms requires concordance. The best practice suggests that the clinician first targets those symptoms the patient finds most distressing. That being said, attempts to stabilize

510

| Therapy | Treatment Course | Gestalt |
|---|---|---|
| Cognitive Behavioral Therapy (CBT) | 8–16 weekly sessions | The goal of trauma-focused CBT is to prevent patients from avoiding their traumatic memories by confronting their disruptive thought patterns[39] |
| Prolonged Exposure Therapy (PE) | 15 weekly sessions over a 3-mo period | PE is a manualized trauma-focused psychotherapy that focuses on imaginal exposure whereby patients recount their traumatic narrative out loud repeatedly.[34] In conjunction with recounting the narrative, in vivo exposure and emotional processing occurs |
| Cognitive Processing Therapy (CPT) | 8–10 90-min sessions over a 6-wk period | CPT is a manualized therapy that combines written exercises with cognitive therapy. During this trauma-focused therapy, patients write about their worst traumatic event, read it back to the therapist, and process their emotions.[40] Patients read their traumatic event daily and during each session the therapist uses Socratic questioning to challenge cognitive distortions. Later, patients challenge their beliefs about the trauma, self, and others[40] |
| Eye Movement Desensitization and Reprocessing (EMDR) | 1–2 times per week for a total of 6–12 sessions | EMDR involves both exposure and cognitive therapy with the addition of external bilateral stimulation. Typically, the stimulation is in the form of eye movements. EMDR is effective in reducing negative emotions and arousal in addition to reducing depression and anxiety in PTSD patients.[41] EMDR's 3-part protocol includes processing traumatic events that have created dysfunction to associate new adaptive information, target distressful circumstances to desensitize internal and external triggers, and incorporate imaginal templates or prospective events for adaptive functioning[42] |
| Brief Eclectic Psychotherapy (BEP) | 16 60-min weekly sessions | BEP is a psychodynamic therapy that incorporates imaginal exposure, written narrative, and cognitive processing to assist the patient in leaving the traumatic event in the past and gain a sense of control.[34] The psychodynamic component of BEP focuses on the emotions of shame and guilt and the therapeutic relationship of the patient and therapist[43] |

**Table 4**
**Informed psychotherapeutic treatment of trauma**

(continued on next page)

| Therapy | Treatment Course | Gestalt |
|---------|------------------|---------|
| **Table 4**<br>**(continued)** | | |
| Adaptive Disclosure Therapy (ADT) | 8 90-min weekly sessions | A specific form of CBT that focuses psychotherapeutic effort on war zone experiences (eg, life threat, traumatic loss, moral injury, and the violation of closely held beliefs or codes) intent to generate moral repair |
| Narrative Exposure Therapy (NET) | 4–10 sessions | Patients create a coherent chronologic narrative of their life story, enabling them to reflect on their entire life and to contextualize their traumatic experience |

*Data from* Refs.[34,39–43]

sleep early can have a significant effect on other trauma symptoms. The use of as-needed pro re nata (PRN) agents such as gabapentin, hydroxyzine, and propranolol can serve as an effective rescue medication for anxiety provided that the patient is benzodiazepine naive. The use of propranolol is particularly useful in those situations where a patient can anticipate a trigger and take it ahead of exposure. Although hydroxyzine is commonly used for anxiety, its antihistaminergic properties can yield marked sedation, which can impair functioning. Alternatively, gabapentin boasts fairly decent anxiolytic properties and is renally excreted, and subsequently caries a low risk for self-harm. Buspirone boasts anxiolytic properties but, like its antidepressant brethren, requires weeks of titration to generate a clinically significant response. Buspirone requires twice-daily dosing and should never be used as a PRN agent. Although both the SSRI (selective serotonin reuptake inhibitors) and SNRI (serotonin-norepinephrine reuptake inhibitors) drug classifications have demonstrated benefit in treating trauma-spectrum symptoms, only sertraline, paroxetine, and venlafaxine carry the FDA indication. Although both classes of antidepressants boast robust side-effect profiles, it is incumbent on the prescribing provider to choose the best possible agent mindful of its side-effect profile and the patient's history. Prazosin has been on the market for decades as an α-blocker for the treatment of hypertension and benign prostatic hyperplasia. It is only in the past couple of decades that its benefits have been identified with traumatic nightmares. Dosing strategies and guidelines can be found in *Stahl's Prescriber's Guide*, 6th Edition.[46]

### Tomorrow's trauma informed treatment
Much has been said recently about new candidates for the treatment of trauma-spectrum symptoms. Accelerated Resolution Therapy (ART) has recently generated some energy in the profession. Using strategies similar to PE and eye movement desensitization and reprocessing, ART aspires to change the way in which negative images are stored in the brain. Although the early evidence is encouraging, ART does not yet have sufficient evidentiary support to stand alongside CPT or PE at this time.[47] A manualized MDMA (3,4-methylenedioxymethamphetamine)-assisted form of psychotherapy is currently in phase 3 trials with the FDA for severe PTSD. The early evidence suggests that MDMA may increase activation in the prefrontal cortex (activation) and decrease activation in the amygdala.[48-50] Although new treatments of PTSD are encouraging, until such time

**Table 5**
**Pharmacopeia for trauma-related and stressor-related disorders**

| Drug Classification | Dosing Range | Mechanism of Action |
|---|---|---|
| *Antidepressant Agents* | | |
| Selective serotonin reuptake inhibitors (SSRI)<br>• Sertraline (Zoloft) *FDA*<br>• Paroxetine (Paxil) *FDA* | • 50–200 mg QD<br>• 20–60 mg QD | Increases serotonin output in both the amygdala-centered and cortico-striato-thalamo-cortical (CTSC) circuits, thereby targeting fear and worry, respectively[39] |
| Serotonin-norepinephrine reuptake inhibitors (SNRI)<br>• Venlafaxine (Effexor XR) *FDA* | • 37.5–225 mg QD | Increases serotonin and norepinephrine output in both the amygdala-centered and CTSC circuits, thereby targeting fear and worry, respectively[39] |
| *Anxiolytic Agents* | | |
| Alpha 2 delta ligand ($\alpha2\delta$L)<br>• Gabapentin (Neurontin) *EBP* | • 100–300 mg PO TID PRN anxiety | Blocks the release of excitatory neurotransmitter glutamate at voltage-sensitive calcium channels in both the amygdala-centered and CTSC circuits[44] |
| Histamine receptor antagonist (H-Ran)<br>• Hydroxyzine (Atarax) *EBP* | • 50–100 mg PO TID to QID PRN anxiety | Block of $H_1$ receptors yielding sedative properties and the suppression of certain subcortical regions of the brain[40] |
| $5HT_{1A}$ partial agonist (SPA)<br>• Buspirone (BuSpar) *FDA* | • 7.5–30 mg PO BID | Targets $5HT_{1A}$ receptor subtypes in presynaptic autoreceptors in the raphe nucleus and postsynaptic heteroreceptors in the limbic system[39] |
| *$\alpha$1-Adrenergic Blocker* | | |
| Selective $\alpha$1-adrenergic receptor antagonist<br>• Prazosin (Minipress) *EBP* | • 1–16 mg PO QHS | $\alpha$1-Adrenergic receptor antagonism leads to smooth muscle relaxation in the peripheral vasculature, which may also contribute to a blockade of postsynaptic $\alpha$-adrenoceptors[41] |
| *$\beta_{1,2}$-Adrenoreceptor Antagonist* | | |
| • Propranolol (Inderal LA) *EBP* | • 60–240 mg PO QD | Binds to $\beta$-adrenoreceptors, thereby blocking the binding of norepinephrine and epinephrine and attenuating sympathetic nervous system (eg, fight or flight) activation[42] |

*Abbreviations:* BID, twice daily; *EBP*, evidence-based support; *FDA*, FDA indicated; PO, by mouth; PRN, pro re nata; QD, daily; QHS, nightly at bedtime; TID, 3 times daily.
    *Data from* Refs.[39–42,44]

that they meet the evidence-based practice bar, health care providers are better served by becoming more adept at leveraging what is already established in the evidence-based armamentarium.

## IMPLICATIONS FOR NURSING

The unquestioned advances in nursing from the likes of Nightingale, Dix, Breckinridge, Barton, and Wald were not born of hubris but, rather, unmitigated social need. It is argued that nursing stands at the precipice of social need once again. There are inadequate resources available to address the demand for evidence-based and trauma informed veteran care. There are currently millions of veterans trying to find their way home. The goal of this article is to provide those clinicians interested in delivering care to this population with a basic set of guidelines to practice intent to help them get home.

## REFERENCES

1. Homer. The iliad. New York: Barnes and Noble Books; 2004.
2. Cohen SP, Brown C, Kurihanara C, et al. Diagnoses and factors associated with medical evacuation and return to duty for service members participating in Operation Iraqi Freedom or Operation Enduring Freedom: a prospective cohort study. Lancet 2010;375(9711):301–9.
3. Goodman GP, DeZee KJ, Burks R, et al. Epidemiology of psychiatric disorders sustained by a U.S. Army brigade combat team during the Iraq War. Gen Hosp Psychiatry 2011;33(1):51–7.
4. Armed Forces Health Surveillance Center. Medical surveillance monthly report. Silver Spring (MD): Armed Forces Health Surveillance Center; 2012.
5. Pruitt LD, Smolenski DJ, Bush NE, et al. Department of defense suicide event report (DoDSER) calendar year 2016 annual report. National Center for Telehealth and Technology (T2) Joint Base Lewis-McChord; 2018.
6. United States Census Bureau. American community survey 2016. Available at. https://www.census.gov/programs-surveys/acs/news/data-releases/2016.html.
7. Kilpatrick DG, Resnick HS, Milanak ME, et al. National estimates of exposure to traumatic events and PTSD prevalence using DSM-IV and DSM-5 criteria. J Trauma Stress 2013;26(5):537–47.
8. Kessler RC, Sonnega A, Bromet E, et al. Posttraumatic stress disorder in the National Comorbidity Survey. Arch Gen Psychiatry 1995;52(12):1048–60.
9. Perkonigg A, Kessler RC, Storz S, et al. Traumatic events and post-traumatic stress disorder in the community: prevalence, risk factors and comorbidity. Acta Psychiatr Scand 2000;101(1):46–59.
10. Neylan TC, Marmar CR, Metzler TJ, et al. Sleep disturbances in the Vietnam generation: findings from a nationally representative sample of male Vietnam veterans. Am J Psychiatry 1998;155(7):929–33.
11. Schlenger WE, Kulka RA, Fairbank JA, et al. The prevalence of post-traumatic stress disorder in the Vietnam generation: a multimethod, multisource assessment of psychiatric disorder. J Trauma Stress 1992;5(3):333–63.
12. Richardson LK, Frueh BC, Acierno R. Prevalence estimates of combat-related post-traumatic stress disorder: critical review. Aust N Z J Psychiatry 2010;44(1):4–19.
13. Litz BT, Schlenger WE. PTSD in service members and new veterans of the Iraq and Afghanistan wars: a bibliography and critique. PTSD Res Q 2009;20(1):1–7.
14. Iverson AC, Fear NT, Ehlers A, et al. Risk factors for post traumatic stress disorder among UK armed forces personnel. Psychol Med 2008;38:1–12.
15. Phillips CJ, Leardmann CA, Gumbs GR, et al. Risk factors for posttraumatic stress disorder among deployed US male marines. BMC Psychiatry 2010;10:52.

16. Seal KH, Metzler TJ, Gima KS, et al. Trends and risk factors for mental health diagnosis among Iraq and Afghanistan veterans using Department of Veterans Affairs health care, 2002-2008. Am J Public Health 2009;99(9):1651–8.

17. Shen YC, Arkes J, Kwan BW, et al. Effects of Iraq/Afghanistan deployments on PTSD diagnoses for still active personnel in all four services. Mil Med 2010; 175(10):763–9.

18. American Psychiatric Association. Diagnostic and statistical manual of mental disorders (DSM-5®). American Psychiatric Association Publishing; 2013.

19. Kessler RC, Chiu WT, Demler O, et al. Prevalence, severity, and comorbidity of 12-month DSM-IV disorders in the National Comorbidity Survey Replication. Arch Gen Psychiatry 2005;62(6):617–27.

20. Goldstein RB, Smith SM, Chou SP, et al. The epidemiology of DSM-5 posttraumatic stress disorder in the United States: results from the National Epidemiologic Survey on Alcohol and Related Conditions—III. Soc Psychiatry Psychiatr Epidemiol 2016;51(8):1137–48.

21. Breslau N. Epidemiologic studies of trauma, posttraumatic stress disorder, and other psychiatric disorders. Los Angeles (CA): SAGE Publications; 2002.

22. Brewin CR, Andrews B, Valentine JD. Meta-analysis of risk factors for posttraumatic stress disorder in trauma-exposed adults. J Consult Clin Psychol 2000; 68(5):748–66.

23. Abdallah CG, Southwick SM, Krystal JH. Neurobiology of posttraumatic stress disorder (PTSD): a path from novel pathophysiology to innovative therapeutics. Neurosci Lett 2017;649:130–2.

24. Belleville G, Guay S, Marchand A. Impact of sleep disturbances on PTSD symptoms and perceived health. J Nerv Ment Dis 2009;197(2):126–32.

25. Cukor J, Wyka K, Mello B, et al. The longitudinal course of PTSD among disaster workers deployed to the World Trade Center following the attacks of September 11th. J Trauma Stress 2011;24(5):506–14.

26. Chopra MP, Zhang H, Pless Kaiser A, et al. PTSD is a chronic, fluctuating disorder affecting the mental quality of life in older adults. Am J Geriatr Psychiatry 2014; 22(1):86–97.

27. Lamarche LJ, De Koninck J. Sleep disturbance in adults with posttraumatic stress disorder: a review. J Clin Psychiatry 2007;68(8):1257–70.

28. Leskin GA, Woodward SH, Yough HE, et al. Effects of comorbid diagnoses on sleep disturbance in PTSD. J Psychiatr Res 2002;36(6):449–52.

29. Ohayon MM, Shapiro CM. Sleep disturbances and psychiatric disorders associated with posttraumatic stress disorder in the general population. Compr Psychiatry 2000;41(6):469–78.

30. Koren D, Arnon I, Lavie P, et al. Sleep complaints as early predictors of posttraumatic stress disorder: a 1-year prospective study of injured survivors of motor vehicle accidents. Am J Psychiatry 2002;159(5):855–7.

31. Machtinger EL, Cuca YP, Khanna N, et al. From treatment to healing: the promise of trauma-informed primary care. Womens Health Issues 2015;25(3):193–7.

32. Oral R, Ramirez M, Coohey C, et al. Adverse childhood experiences and trauma informed care: the future of health care. Pediatr Res 2015;79(1–2):227.

33. Raja S, Hasnain M, Hoersch M, et al. Trauma informed care in medicine. Fam Community Health 2015;38(3):216–26.

34. The Management of Posttraumatic Stress Disorder Work Group. VA/DoD clinical practice guideline for the management of posttraumatic stress disorder and acute stress disorder. Department of Veterans Affairs. Department of Defense. Version 3.0. 2017; 33–34.

35. Steenkamp MM, Litz BT, Hoge CW, et al. Psychotherapy for military-related PTSD: a review of randomized clinical trials. JAMA 2015;314(5):489–500.

36. Maguen S, Madden E, Cohen BE, et al. Time to treatment among veterans of conflicts in Iraq and Afghanistan with psychiatric diagnoses. Psychiatr Serv 2012; 63(12):1206–12.

37. Hembree EA, Foa EB, Dorfan NM, et al. Do patients drop out prematurely from exposure therapy for PTSD? J Trauma Stress 2003;16(6):555–62.

38. Schottenbauer MA, Glass CR, Arnkoff DB, et al. Nonresponse and dropout rates in outcome studies on PTSD: review and methodological considerations. Psychiatry 2008;71(2):134–68.

39. Stahl SM. Stahl's essential psychopharmacology: neuroscientific basis and practical application. 4th edition. New York: Cambridge University Press; 2013.

40. Dowben JS, Grant JS, Froelich KD, et al. Biological perspectives: hydroxyzine for anxiety: another look at an old drug. Perspect Psychiatr Care 2013;49(2):75–7.

41. George KC, Kebejian L, Ruth LJ, et al. Meta-analysis of the efficacy and safety of prazosin versus placebo for the treatment of nightmares and sleep disturbances in adults with posttraumatic stress disorder. J Trauma Dissociation 2016;17(4): 494–510.

42. Gorre F, Vandekerckhove H. Beta-blockers: focus on mechanism of action. Which beta-blocker, when and why? Acta Cardiol 2010;65(5):565–70.

43. Stahl SM. Prescriber's guide, children and adolescents: Stahl's essential psychopharmacology. New York: Cambridge University Press; 2018.

44. Houghton KT, Forrest A, Awad A, et al. Biological rationale and potential clinical use of gabapentin and pregabalin in bipolar disorder, insomnia and anxiety: protocol for a systematic review and meta-analysis. BMJ Open 2017;7(3):e013433.

45. Axmon A, Kristensson J, Ahlstrom G, et al. Use of antipsychotics, benzodiazepine derivatives, and dementia medication among older people with intellectual disability and/or autism spectrum disorder and dementia. Res Dev Disabil 2017;62:50–7.

46. Stahl SM. Stahl's essential psychopharmacology: prescriber's guide. 6th edition. New York: Cambridge University Press; 2017.

47. Waits W, Marumoto M, Weaver J. Accelerated resolution therapy (ART): a review and research to date. Curr Psychiatry Rep 2017;19(3):18.

48. Slomski A. MDMA-assisted psychotherapy for PTSD. JAMA 2018;319(24):2470.

49. Feduccia AA, Mithoefer MC. MDMA-assisted psychotherapy for PTSD: are memory reconsolidation and fear extinction underlying mechanisms? Prog Neuropsychopharmacol Biol Psychiatry 2018;84(Pt A):221–8.

50. Sessa B. MDMA and PTSD treatment: "PTSD: from novel pathophysiology to innovative therapeutics". Neurosci Lett 2017;649:176–80.

# Management of Attention-Deficit/Hyperactivity Disorder in Primary Care

Kathleen T. McCoy, DNSc, APRN, PMHNP-BC, PMHCNS-BC, FNP-BC[a],
Kirsten Pancione, DNP, PMHNP-BC, FNP-BC[a],
Linda Sue Hammonds, DNP, PMHNP-BC, FNP[a],
Christine B. Costa, DNP, PMHNP-BC[b,*]

## KEYWORDS

- Attention-deficit/hyperactivity disorder (ADHD) • Risk factors • Comorbidities
- Family dynamics • Level of function (LoF) • Genetic predisposition
- Pharmacogenetics • Holistic care

## KEY POINTS

- Attention-deficit/hyperactivity disorder (ADHD) presentations are global, across the life span with diverse features.
- Patients prefer primary care settings to psychiatric settings for management of ADHD, with primary care providing the majority of pharmacologic treatment.
- Undiagnosed and/or untreated ADHD presents myriad risks to personal and public health.
- ADHD is highly genetic, with family impact/dynamics management essential to enhance recovery in a holistic manner.
- Comorbidities are common, requiring timely, accurate diagnosis and adequate care.

## INTRODUCTION

Attention-deficit/hyperactivity disorder (ADHD) can be defined as a mental disorder that affects the ability to discriminate between stimuli to a point that it affects functionality in 2 or more areas (social, intellectual, work life, etc.)[1] ADHD is a global issue, with prevalence rating between 1% and 20% according to a meta-analysis by Polanczyk and colleagues.[2] Global results are limited due to incongruence

Disclosure Statement: No disclosures.
[a] Department of Community Mental Health, University of South Alabama, College of Nursing, HAHN 304 / 5721 USA Drive North, Mobile, AL 36688-002, USA; [b] California State University, Long Beach, School of Nursing, 1250 Bellflower Boulevard, MS 0301, Long Beach, CA 90804, USA
* Corresponding author.
*E-mail address:* christine.costa@csulb.edu

Nurs Clin N Am 54 (2019) 517–532
https://doi.org/10.1016/j.cnur.2019.08.001
0029-6465/19/Published by Elsevier Inc.

between diagnostic criteria, globally. See the current diagnostic requirements according to the *Diagnostic and Statistical Manual of Mental Disorders* (Fifth Edition) (*DSM-5*),[1] which detail the diagnostic criteria for ADHD. The continuous patterns of inattention and/or hyperactivity impeding the level of functioning and/or developmental progression for minimum of 6 months to a degree not in keeping with appropriate developmental milestone negatively affecting function remains unchanged, with mild, moderate, or severe presentations.[1] Primarily, there is little difference between the United States and Europe; however, beyond these 2 geographic areas, there are numerous differences, including levels of functionality. For this reason, this article is limited to a discussion of ADHD in primary care (PC) settings in the United States, where prevalence, incidence, and treatment options have increased in the past decade.[2]

## ETIOLOGY

The growing body of literature does not affirm simple linear causal pathways in which a single genetic and/or environmental risk leads to a single cognitive deficit sufficient to cause all symptoms of disorders, such as ADHD, reading disorders, and/or mathematics disabilities. Developmental disorders, including ADHD, are better conceptualized as heterogeneous conditions arising from additive and interactive effects, including both genetic and environmental risk factors. Furthermore, high heritability, especially concerning dopamine (D) pathways, led to initial optimism that genes with major effects could be identified for ADHD. This rendered etiologies to be complex, polygenetic, and with multiple genetic/environment risks. Environmental risks include prenatal alcohol use, smoking, toxin exposure, brain injuries, low birth weight, postnatal being socioeconomic status, and environmental adversity implicating the stress diathesis model. Combined risks contribute to total phenotypic variance in this population. The confluence of current literature argues vigorously against single-gene models, leading to a consensus that more research is required to better understand ADHD causation.[3,4]

## INCIDENCE

The global proportion of population prevalence of ADHD is between 2% and 20%, per the World Health Organization, in 2015.[5] There is no global consensus, however, for criteria for diagnosis and impact of variances in level of function. Therefore, the statistics move positively in which criteria are clear with functionality addressed, and vice versa, in part, explaining the wide global spread in prevalence. The *Summary Health Statistics for U.S. Children: National Health Interview Survey, 2011*, correlated the 2010 US Census, soon due for 2020 US Census update.[6] The 2010 US Census used the then-current *Diagnostic and Statistical Manual of Mental Disorders* (Fourth Edition, Text Revision),[7] and noted inclusion as aggregate data, all types of recognized ADHD (inattentive, hyperactive, and mixed types). The following data correlations include children with ADHD with stable 2-parent families, whose parents exceed high school diplomas, who have robust socioeconomic status, who possess health insurance and receive more regular health care, who take medicine more regularly, and who lose fewer days off from school due to injury/illness. Children with ADHD in poverty, in less stable households, and who are uninsured or underinsured and may not see a provider or see a provider in a timely manner may not take medicine with regularity and may lose more time off from school due to illness/injury. See **Table 1** for additional 2010 US Census/ ADHD-related correlates.

| Table 1 |
|---|
| Attention-deficit/hyperactivity disorder characteristics, incidence, and prevalence (United States) |

| US Children Population: Year 2011 | Descriptors: Age 3–17 |
|---|---|
| LD, including ADHD | Total 4.7 million children (8%)<br>Boys: 9%<br>Girls: 8% |
| Race and presence of LD | White: 8%<br>Black: 9%<br>Asian: 5% |
| Income <$35,000 | 11% |
| Income >$100,000 | 5% |
| ADHD | Exceeds 5 million children<br>Boys: 12%<br>Girls: 5% |
| Race prevalence | Hispanic: 6%<br>Non-Hispanic white:10%<br>Non-Hispanic black: 9% |
| Single-mother families | LD: 10%<br>ADHD: 10% |
| Two-parent families | LD: 6%<br>ADHD: 8% |
| Excellent/very good health status | LD: 6%<br>ADHD: 7% |
| Fair/poor health status | LD: 38% (7-fold increase over excellent/very good health status)<br>ADHD: 27% (4-fold increase over excellent/very good health status) |
| Prescription medication use | 14% of US children endorse medicine regularity in last 3 mo<br>Boys: 15%<br>Girls: 12% |
| Percentage of children on regular medicine: age group | 12–17 y: 18%<br>5–11 y: 13%<br>4 years/under: 9% |

*Abbreviation:* LD, learning disability.
*Data from* Bloom, RA Cohen, G Freeman. Summary health statistics for U.S. children: National Health Interview Survey, 2011. National Center for Health Statistics. Vital Health Stat. 2012; 10(254).

## PATHOPHYSIOLOGY AND THEORY

Currently, the pathogenesis of ADHD is not conclusively known. Stahl[8] posits ADHD to be linked to arousal mechanism neurobiology, with hyperactive children being over aroused/overstimulated. Defective inhibitory mechanisms of the neurodevelopmentally compromised prefrontal cortex may contribute to insufficient information processes, resulting in ADHD symptoms of inattention, hyperactivity, and impulsivity. Agents increasing the arousal drive network, by enhancing D and norepinephrine (NE) synaptic actions can improve efficacy of information processing in the prefrontal circuits, and paradoxically improve ADHD symptoms, moving arousal from deficient to normal. The hypoactive brain associated with ADHD (inattention) is likewise associated with decreased frequency of tonic firing of D and NE neurons. Deficient arousal mechanisms can be increased to normal activation levels with stimulants and with the

NE transporter network inhibitors. Persons with ADHD are generally unable to activate prefrontal cortex areas correctly in response to cognitive tasks of attention and executive function. Some persons may be unable to activate the dorsal anterior cingulate cortex, recruiting other brain regions to accomplish tasks, being slower and subject to error. When treated with agents activating D, cognitive ability increases. There are links to sleep centers as well, causing sleepiness, lethargy, or, conversely, hyperarousal and may result in sleep cycle disturbances. Treatment with stimulants relieves ADHD symptoms, causing normal firing rates of both D and NE neurons, which can be linked to normal arousal and efficient information processing in the prefrontal cortex, resulting in normal levels of attention, motor activity, and impulse control. With low mechanisms of arousal, pyramid neurons in the prefrontal cortex are not in sync and unable to distinguish important neuronal signals from unimportant ones. When this happens, people are unable to focus on 1 thing more than another because all signals are perceived as the same because attention is unsustained, and distraction occurs between signals, resulting in thoughtless movement/impulsive action. Increasing prefrontal arousal mechanisms by enhancing D and NE activity may improve signal-to-noise ability in the prefrontal cortex, relieving ADHD symptoms. D acting on certain D receptors may diminish levels of noise, and NE, acting at $\alpha_{2A}$-adrenergic receptors, may improve the signal size. The idea of malfunctioning perceptual circuits being out-of-tune, rather than too high or low, is another issue operating in the treatment of ADHD.[7] Increasingly, there is focus on ADHD and the genetic role. See **Box 1** for genetic influences.

## SOCIAL DETERMINANTS OF HEALTH AND EFFECTS ON HEALTH AND SAFETY

Readers are referred to **Box 2** for inferences closely linked to social determinants of health: ADHD characteristics, incidence, and prevalence in the United States. Awareness of intersecting effects of race, gender, family constitution, social support, and socioeconomic status on ADHD is important.[11,12] For example, whether income operates as a risk or protective factor for ADHD patients depends on race, gender, and other socioeconomic characteristics, including family constellation and type of health insurance coverage. Therefore, frameworks created to incorporate social determinants of health provide a more complete picture of the extent to which patients and their families respond to ADHD and what it takes to readily access quality health care, targeted to individual and family related health outcomes.

---

**Box 1**
**Genetic influences**

- Genes appearing to play a role in the development of ADHD have shown in monozygotic twins at 92% and in dizygotic twins 33%[9]
- Dopamine D2, D4, and D5 receptor genes (DRD2, DRD4, and DRD5)
- Serotonin transporter genes (SLC6A3 and SLC6A4)
- Serotonin 1B receptor gene (HTR1B)
- Dopamine beta-hydroxylase gene (DBH)
- Synaptosome associated protein 25 kDa (SNAP25)
- Glutamate receptors, metabotropic (GRM1, GRM5, GRM7, and GRM8)
- Prenatal exposure to maternal (viral/smoke/stress/malnutrition)[5,10]

*Data from* Refs.[5,9,10]

---

---

**Box 2**
**Social determinant screening**

Social: adverse childhood experiences, poor education, and food insecurity

Environmental: poor housing quality, family instability, unemployment, and discrimination

Health-related behaviors: poor eating, excessive drinking and substance use, smoking, physical inactivity, and recklessness (including driving and impulsive behavior)

*Data from* Kaufman JS. Causal Inference for Social Exposures Annual Review of Public Health Commentary. *Public Health Rev.* 2018;39:19.

---

Screening for ADHD and social determinants of health help identify patients potentially benefiting from greater support in one or more areas. Screening promotes a holistic, public health approach, especially for the marginalized and underserved, factors closely linked to health outcomes. Evidence supports social screening and early intervention in primary care, while recognizing the need to continue developing and refining available screening tools and interventions. Screening for social determinants of mental health includes but is not limited to identifying factors, such as family history of psychiatric illness, adverse early life experiences, unemployment, food insecurity, homelessness/housing instability, and domestic/intimate partner violence coupled with a more complete health history. Screening for social determinants of health in clinical care helps to move the marginalized closer to the mainstream.[10]

Policy changes to address social determinants of health, such as poverty, racism, violence, and access to resources, can have a far-reaching impact on improving the health of a community, state or country. Andermann[13] states although there are no universal screening requirements for social determinants, addressing only symptoms and ignoring root causes do not improve population health. Screening benefits include providing whole-person care, improved diagnostic accuracy by having all the important information in terms of living conditions and social context, decreased costs by early intervention, increased adherence to treatment regimens, and structurally competent care.[13]

## GENERAL POPULATION PRESENTATION OF ATTENTION-DEFICIT/HYPERACTIVITY DISORDER

There are differing variations of ADHD, as evidenced by diagnostic qualifiers, as well as degrees of functional impairment. ADHD is the focus of this article, with typical presentations examined. Being genetically linked, family members presenting with co-occurring disorders are to be considered for appropriate therapeutic management. Other high-risk populations vulnerable to include those with substance abuse, those who are pregnant, the elderly, adolescents, and young adults in academically pressured environments. It is important to carefully consider differential diagnosis and gather a thorough history with pertinent information about behavioral issues, questions, and observations using *DSM-5* diagnostic criteria, including medication history and review.[1] Screening and treatment should include growth/weight history, current symptom presentation, and level of functional impairments. See **Table 2** provides an overview of common co-occurring disorders, screening considerations, and treatment approaches.

The presentations of ADHD varies across the life span. Therefore, symptoms need to be viewed in context of capacity to impair function for expected developmental level, most often related to academics or employment functioning. The initial plan of

**Table 2**
**Overview of attention-deficit/hyperactivity disorder common co-occurring disorders, screening, and treatment approaches**

| Diagnosis/ Symptoms | Screening | Treatment Considerations/Approaches |
|---|---|---|
| Mood disorders | Pediatric Symptom Checklist-17 for ages 4–17 (filled out by parent/child)[14,15]<br>PHQ-9: modified for teens for over the age 11[16]<br>Mood Disorder Questionnaire-9[17] | Individuals with mood disorders should be screened for ADHD, which occurs at a substantially higher rate among those with mood disorders than the general population[18] |
| Substance use | Alcohol Use Disorders Identification Test[19]<br>CAGE questionnaire[20]<br>Drug screen lottery | • Monitor medicine: parental/ school nurse<br>• Inquire about substance use for all adolescents<br>• State drug log review |
| Pregnancy | β-HCG | • Inquire<br>  ○ Last menstrual period<br>  ○ Intimate contact<br>  ○ Active family<br>  ○ planning |
| Other learning disorders | Thorough history pertinent to learning disorder in question[1] | • Referral: diagnostic testing<br>• Collaborate with school district contact |
| Oppositional defiance | Identification of oppositional defiant behavior for effective treatment[21] | Collaboration:<br>• Case worker<br>• School district liaison<br>• Other stakeholders |
| Sleep disorders | Identification of sleep disorders that are common in ADHD[22] | • Sleep hygiene inventory (screen)<br>• Sleep log<br>• Referral sleep specialist/ neurology<br>• Caffeine intake monitoring |
| Tics | Thorough history pertinent to behavioral issue/s[1]<br>Observation | • Remove offending agent<br>• Neurology consult |
| Seizures | Thorough history pertinent to behavioral issue/s[1]<br>Observation | • Remove offending agent<br>• Seizure log<br>• Neurology collaboration |
| Cardiac | Thorough history pertinent to behavioral issue/s[1]<br>Observation | • ECG[23]<br>• Coordination of care with cardiology/pediatrics<br>• Medication adjustment to medications with reduced cardiac risk |
| Pregnancy | β-HCG | • Weigh risk vs benefits when using pharmacologic agents[24] |
| Anorexia | Thorough history pertinent to behavioral issue/s[1]<br>Observation weight/girth q visit | • Remove agent/s attenuating condition<br>• Nutritional consult/follow-up<br>• Family therapy |

(continued on next page)

| Table 2 (continued) | | |
|---|---|---|
| **Diagnosis/ Symptoms** | **Screening** | **Treatment Considerations/Approaches** |
| Growth disorders | Thorough history pertinent to behavioral issue/s[1] <br> Observation <br> Weight/height, every visit | • Referral endocrinology <br> • Risk vs benefit decision with family/patient <br> • Remove agents attenuating condition <br> • Consider summers and weekends as medication off-times |

*Abbreviations*: HCG, human chorionic gonadotropin; PHQ, Patient Heath Questionnaire.
   *Data from* Refs.[1,14–24]

care considers Americans with Disabilities Act (ADA) accommodations that may need to be filed with school/employment. It then is critical to ascertain the level of available support.[25] Family systems theory has implications for all persons in close proximity or residing with and/or dependent on the family system to assist level of function to be optimal. This is especially important when treating preschool/school-aged children to accurately assess response to medication and follow through environmental recommendations with identified family and/or support systems.[26,27] See **Table 3** for screening and treatment considerations across the life span.

## CLINICAL TREATMENT GOAL: RECOVERY AND REMISSION OF SYMPTOMS

ADHD is a treatable, lifelong condition with many paths to recovery and/or a remitted/enhanced state of health and stability of being with optimal function in all spheres. As a biological state, true remission requires holistic approaches, known now as multimodal therapy, that is specific to each individual and family, extending beyond primary care environments of care and incorporating social/spiritual needs, academic augmentation, and employment adjustments as a lifelong dynamic in care approaches, changing developmentally across life span trajectories. This approach may be enhanced or require a case/care manager at all or select times and is best facilitated in an integrated care practice. It is expected that symptoms fluidly wax and wane depending on people's changing life circumstances and functional expectations.[27,28]

## DISCUSSION

The following treatment issues remain in ever-present clinical dialogue.

### Safety

Bonham[37] expressed valid concerns surrounding ADHD, mostly about impulsivity and poor judgment. These concerns include motor vehicle, traffic, and other injuries, including occupational injuries as well as unintended pregnancy.[36,37] In a 2017 *JAMA* publication, in a national cohort study exceeding 2 million patients with ADHD, therapeutic medication was associated with a significant reduction in the risk of motor vehicle crashes in both men and women.[36] This finding supports medicine as a mitigation strategy for risk, injury, and other results and is, therefore, is worth considering as a daily habit, regardless of the presence/absence of a school day or work day.

**Table 3**
Across life span attention-deficit/hyperactivity disorder clinical presentation/screens/
evidence-informed approaches

| Population | Screening | Considerations | Treatments/ Pharmacology |
|---|---|---|---|
| Pediatric | Vanderbilt Screen for home/school<br>Thorough history elicitation, home and school<br>1. Vanderbilt initial assessment (Parent administered)<br>2. Vanderbilt initial assessment (Teacher administered)<br>3. Vanderbilt follow up (Parent administered)<br>4. Vanderbilt follow up (Teacher administered)[28]<br>Screen for child anxiety-related disorders using SCARED[29–31]<br>Pediatric Symptom Checklist for ages 4–17[32]<br>PHQ-9[32]<br>ADHD Rating Scale-IV validated for preschool children)[33] | Dietary influences, food additives, refined sugar, food sensitivity, essential fatty acids, iron deficiency, zinc deficiency<br>With stimulant class: Baseline ECG[23]<br>Family considerations<br>Positive reinforcement<br>Differentials for anxiety and bipolar which may mimic ADHD symptoms[33] | Behavior therapy, including training for parents:<br>Create a routine<br>Get organized<br>Manage distractions<br>Limit choices<br>Be clear/specific when speaking with your child<br>Help your child plan<br>Use realistic goals and praise or other rewards<br>Track positive behaviors<br>Discipline effectively<br>Create positive opportunities.<br>Provide a healthy lifestyle[31,33]<br>School accommodations and interventions[25,31]<br>Multimodal therapies[25–27]<br>Medications[23,33]<br>Stimulants:<br>• Amphetamine<br>• Lidexamphetamine<br>• Amphetamine/ dextroamphetamine<br>• Dextroamphetamine<br>• Methylphenidate<br>• Dexmethylphenidate<br>Nonstimulants:<br>• Atomoxetine<br>• Clonidine<br>• Guanfacine<br>• Bupropion<br>• Venlafaxine[33]<br>(With Food and Drug Administration trials currently requesting ages 4–5 y)[34]<br>Numerous medication vehicles currently available |
| Adolescent | Vanderbilt scales[28]<br>Pediatric Symptom Checklist for ages 4–17[31]<br>PHQ-9[32] (Adolescent Depression)<br>ADHD Rating Scale-IV[33] | (See Pediatric)<br>• Family considerations[35]<br>• Medication management[34]<br>• Driving/machinery safety, pregnancy issues[24,36,37] | (See Pediatric)<br>• Behavior therapy, including training for parents<br>• Medications (see Pediatric)[23,34]<br>• School accommodations and interventions[33] |

(continued on next page)

| Table 3 (continued) | | | |
|---|---|---|---|
| **Population** | **Screening** | **Considerations** | **Treatments/ Pharmacology** |
| Adult | Thorough history and symptoms (*DSM-5*)[1] | • Family considerations<br>• Medication management<br>• Driving/machinery safety issues<br>• Positive reinforcement[34,38] | • Medications (see Pediatric)[39] |
| Geriatric | Although older patients are known to have similar symptoms and comorbidities as younger patients with ADHD, there is little evidence to guide assessment and treatment.[40–42] | Family considerations<br>Medication management<br>Driving/machinery safety issues[36]<br>Care with differentials/ comorbidities<br>Positive reinforcement<br>Consistent use of assistive devices (walkers, canes, spectacles, hearing aids) | • Medications (see Pediatric)[39] |

*Abbreviations*: PHQ, Patient Heath Questionnaire; SCARED, screen for child anxiety related disorders.
*Data from* Refs.[1,23–40]

Risks versus benefits are weighed heavily with long-term safety of ADHD medicines for children. Ongoing concerns in the literature regarding treatment include examining growth, cardiac risk, and metabolic matters, among other issues that continue to be followed as current cohorts grow developmentally into adulthood, per the systematic review of Hennison and colleagues[41,42] and ADDUCE (Attention Deficit Hyperactivity Disorder Drugs Use Chronic Effects) consortium prospective study.

### Diversion

Diversion in general persists as a national issue.[43] Increased diversion of stimulants among college-aged students is concerning.[35] Students at risk for diversion include those under academic pressure, cramming, in poverty, those engaging in recreational use and those who desire to do well on concomitant psychological testing motivated for need of or desire for academic setting and class assignment accommodations. Providers are encouraged to be aware of present risks to prevent misuse, diversion and black-market distribution/sale of these medications. Vigilance reading potential misuse or abuse of medication requires judicious follow-through in care of patients, with drug testing as an option. Alternate options to stimulant medications, including atomoxetine, bupropion, and clonidine, may be considered for patients with substance abuse histories. Practice management strategies are essential to providing safe care and require awareness of diversion risk, which necessitates purposeful, well-planned practice management, including the use of state medication monitoring sites and adherence to local/federal guidelines.

### Drug Holidays

Drug holidays, occurring over weekends, holidays, and summer, for children are a subject of avid discussion. Parents and children may prefer days off medicines, yet children and teens may be at risk for untoward and/or high-risk behaviors while on drug holidays. There is no single correct approach, so it is important to maintain flexibility while working with a patient and family on a treatment regimen. As recently as 2018, researchers like Ibrahim and Donyai[44] and Barnard-Brak and colleagues[45] have debated the matter by looking at the reluctance of providers to discuss breaks and adherence breaks.[44,45]

This challenging dialogue occurs within complicated contexts of barriers to treatment as well as new treatment protocols for providers in the effective management of ADHD. These are presented in more detail in **Box 3** and **Table 4**.

## SUMMARY

Recognition and treatment of ADHD in the United States and Europe are in consensus; however, a global broad consensus for definition and degrees of functional

---

**Box 3**
**Current barriers to effective management of attention-deficit/hyperactivity disorder in primary care**

Stigma
  Pervasive to all mental health issues/diagnosis, labels of any psychiatric illness provoke ill-perceived public perceptions and well a legitimate issue with attendant symptoms in vulnerable populations, such as children, adolescents, and adults, in any/all settings, especially school settings where medications may be administered. Stigma is not limited to but includes where persons with ADHD are home, being educated/employed, socializing and when participating in health care.

Current solutions
  Per the *Journal of the American Psychiatric Nurses Association*, Jensen and colleagues[46] call for culture change through broad education, holistic/person-centered language/care approaches and programs, such as *One Voice* and the *LINKS Anti-Stigma* program, for middle managers/front-line leaders as climate setters in organizations likely to treat persons with ADHD.[27,47]

Access to effective care and psychiatric mental health providers:
  Paucity of mental health provider and inadequately prepared primary care providers, especially in rural settings persists. Referrals continue due to lack of provider access. Time management often precludes effective history taking and screening. Reimbursement complexities reward number of encounters rather than quality outcomes.

Current solution/s
  TeleMental-health, MBC, and MIPS.[48–50]

Co-occurring disorders (see **Table 3**)
• Numerous and varied presentations/comorbidities
• Competing demands for clinical time often preclude that which would be spent on adequate history gleaning and differential diagnosis

Solutions:
• MBC screens and thorough history taking[49]
• Integrative care models where somatic and behavioral needs have potential to be treated within one organization[27,38]

Philosophic changes to wellness promoting Centers for Medicare & Medicaid Services initiatives, patient-centered care, holistic and integrative team based approaches, rewarding wellness rather than encounter volume[50]

Solution:
  MIPS, integrative care models[38,50]

*Data from* Refs.[27,38,46–50]

| Table 4 | |
| --- | --- |
| New directions for management of attention-deficit/hyperactivity disorder in primary care | |
| Item/Definition: | Projected Impact |
| Stigma reduction | Education of those impacted by ADHD, caregivers (including family, teachers, clergy, and employers) and public serves to promote more positive ways to accept persons and their families so affected, allowing for better chances of recovery and self-directed lives, bypassing negative and consequential social cues and consequences of rejection, fear, and sanction.[46,47] |
| | ADA accommodations for students and employers help foster recovery while promoting independence and more successful academic and career trajectories.[25] |
| MBC | Adopted as standard of care may transform psychiatric practice, moving mental health patients from fringe to care mainstream, improving access and quality of care, and promoting recovery while reducing economic burden for patients with mental illness by using evidence-informed screens and treatments and team-based care[49] |
| Telehealth access | Telehealth opportunities promote access to care, 24/7, in a variety of supervised settings with increase of numerous third-party payers.[48] |
| Wellness-based reimbursement incentive payment strategies | The Medicare Access and CHIP Reauthorization Act of 2015 passed into law and is a stepping stone to revise Part B Medicare payments, repealing the sustainable growth rate and developing a new payment framework for health care delivery, divided into the MIPS and advanced alternative payment methods. Will become mandatory with bonus incentive payments awarded to practices attaining wellness benchmarks disrupting payment per encounter[50] |

*Abbreviation*: CHIP, Children's Health Insurance Program.
  *Data from* Refs.[25,46–50]

| Box 4 |
| --- |
| Clinical pearls |
| Center for Medicare & Medicaid Systems in process of moving toward adoption of MIPS and wellness initiatives.[50] |
| Reduction of stigma through use of person-first language and stigma-reduction activities promotes respect of patients as persons, decreases stigma, and promotes engagement in self-care.[46,47] |
| Employ patient centeredness, approach patient holistically/integratively, with multimodal approaches family dynamics, psychotherapies, pharmacotherapy, and social, academic, and career aspects of care in mind.[27] |
| Use MBC for efficient screening/diagnostics/treatments and with consideration of plausible differentials/comorbidities at every encounter.[50] |
| Women of childbearing/lactation age to be approached pharmacologically with least teratogenic and/or harmful approaches, with reliable birth control in place, if sexually active when not family planning[24] |
| Use of telehealth and collaborative/integrated care systems best assists patients across the life span, decreasing service gaps and increasing patient/provider satisfaction.[27,48] |
| *Data from* Refs.[24,27,46–48,50] |

impairment is not currently in place.[2] Therefore, this discussion is limited to US populations affected with ADHD. Risks for undiagnosed/untreated ADHD include personal growth and development as well as community liability, including risk to life and limb, social standing, and employment. Public health approaches include increasing access to care, improved care models and reimbursement management, and broad-scale education, including but not limited to stigma-reducing approaches to increase patient participation and reduce bias. ADHD is most often recognized and treated in primary recognition and/or timely effective care places individuals, families, and community settings, by clinicians who may or may not be adequately prepared for its diverse presentations for its multiple personal and public health attendant risks. There are new treatments and approaches based on holistic, patient-centered care, which are outlined in **Box 4**.[27] Providing tools, as in measurement-based care (MBC), and increasing access, through patient-centered/integrative care centers and telehealth and quality incentives, as in Merit-based Incentive Payment System (MIPS), while reducing stigma to encourage patient active health behavior participation may be paving a better path for management of ADHD in primary care settings.[27,46–50]

## REFERENCES

1. American Psychiatric Association. Diagnostic and statistical manual of mental disorders. 5th edition. Washington, DC: American Psychiatric Publishing; 2013. p. 59–61.

2. Polanczyk G, De Lima M, Horta B, et al. The worldwide prevalence of ADHD: a systematic review and metaregression analysis. Am J Psychiatry 2007. https://doi.org/10.1176/appi.ajp.164.6.942.

3. Willcutt EG, Pennington BF, Duncan L, et al. Understanding the complex etiologies of developmental disorders: behavioral and molecular genetic approaches. J Dev Behav Pediatr 2010;31(7):533–44. Available at: https://www.nimh.nih.gov/health/topics/attention-deficit-hyperactivity-disorder-adhd/index.shtml. Accessed December 21, 2018.

4. WHO. Adolescent mental health. 2018. Available at: http://www.who.int/mental_health/maternal-child/adolescent/en/. Accessed November 15, 2018.

5. NIH. Mental health information health topics. Attention deficit 25, hyperactivity disorder. 2016. Webpage. Available at: https://www.nimh.nih.gov/health/topics/attention-deficit-hyperactivity-disorder-adhd/index.shtml. Accessed January 8, 2019.

6. Bloom B, Cohen RA, Freeman G. Summary health statistics for U.S. children: National Health Interview Survey, 2011. Vital Health Stat 10 2012;(254):1–88. National Center for Health Statistics. Available at: https://www.ncbi.nlm.nih.gov/pubmed/25116332. Accessed December 22, 2018.

7. American Psychiatric Association. Diagnostic and statistical manual of mental disorders IV-TR. Washington, DC: American Psychiatric Publishing; 1994.

8. Stahl SM. Stahl's Essential Psychopharmacology: neuroscientific basis and practical application. 3rd edition. Cambridge (United Kingdom): Cambridge University Press; 2008. p. 870–3.

9. Arnsten AFT. The emerging neurobiology of attention deficit hyperactivity disorder: the key role of the prefrontal association cortex. J Pediatr 2009;154(5):I.

10. Lee Y-A, Yamaguchi Y, Goto Y. Neurodevelopmental plasticity in pre- and postnatal environmental interactions: implications for psychiatric disorders from an evolutionary perspective. Neural Plast 2015;2015:9.

11. Sederer LI. The social determinants of mental health. Psychiatr Serv 2016;67(2): 234–5. Available at: https://ps.psychiatryonline.org/doi/10.1176/appi.ps.20150 0232. Accessed December 12, 2018.

12. Behforouz HL, Drain PK, Rhatigan JJ. Rethinking the social history. N Engl J Med 2014;371(14):1277–9. Available at: https://www.nejm.org/doi/full/10.1056/NEJMp 1404846. Accessed December 26, 2018.

13. Andermann A. Screening for social determinants of health in clinical care: moving from the margins to the mainstream. Public Health Rev 2018;39:19. Available at: https:// publichealthreviews.biomedcentral.com/articles/10.1186/s40985-018-0094-7. Accessed January 3, 2019.

14. Murphy JM, Bergmann P, Chiang C, et al. The PSC-17: Subscale Scores, Reliability, and Factor Structure in a New National Sample. Pediatrics 2016; 138(3):e20160038. Available at: http://pediatrics.aappublications.org/content/ pediatrics/early/2016/08/10/peds.2016-0038.full.pdf1515.

15. Gardner W, Murphy M, Childs G, et al. The PSC-17: a brief pediatric symptom checklist with psychosocial problem subscales. A report from PROS and ASPN...Ambulatory Sentinel Practice Network... Pediatric Research in Office Settings... including commentary by Sturner R. Ambul Child Health 1999;5(3): 225–36. Available at: https://libproxy.usouthal.edu/login?url=https://search.ebs cohost.com/login.aspx?direct=true&db=ccm&AN=107096191&site=ehost-live. Accessed November 26, 2018.

16. PHQ-9. PHQ-9: modified for teens and scoring the PHQ-9: modified for teens. 2010. Available at: https://www.aacap.org/App_Themes/AACAP/docs/member_ resources/toolbox_for_clinical_practice_and_outcomes/symptoms/GLAD-PC_PHQ-9.pdf. Accessed January 8, 2019.

17. Tolliver BK, Anton RF. Assessment and treatment of mood disorders in the context of substance abuse. Dialogues Clin Neurosci 2015;17(2):181–90. Available at: https://www.ncbi.nlm.nih.gov/pmc/articles/PMC4518701/. Accessed January 7, 2019.

18. Bond RA, Hadjipavlou G, Lam RW, et al, Canadian Network for Mood and Anxiety Treatments (CANMAT) Task Force. The Canadian Network for Mood and Anxiety Treatments (CANMAT) task force recommendations for the management of patients with mood disorders and comorbid attention deficit hyperactivity disorder. Ann Clin Psychiatry 2012;24:23–37. Available at: https://www.bing.com/search? q=the+canadian+network+for+mood+and+anxiety+treatments+%28canmat %29+task+force+recommendations+for+the+management+of+patients+ with+mood+disorders+and+comorbid+attention-deficit%2Fhyperactivity+dis order.+%2F+bond%2C+david+j.%3B+hadjipavlou%2C+george%3B+lam% 2C+raymond+w.%3B+mcintyre%2C+roger+s.%3B+beaulieu%2C+serge% 3B+schaffer%2C+ayal%3B+weiss%2C+margaret.in%3A+annals+of+clinical +psychiatry%2C+vol.+24%2C+no.+1%2C+0102.2012%2C+p.+23-37.&form =EDGHPT&qs=PF&cvid=814645a07eaa49eeafba19ddbeda44d5&cc=US&set lang=en-US&PC=LCTS.

19. WHO AUDIT(nd) Webpage. Available at: https://www.drugabuse.gov/sites/ default/files/files/AUDIT.pdf. Accessed January 7, 2019.

20. Ewing. CAGE Questionnaire (1984). Webpage. Available at: https://www. hopkinsmedicine.org/johns_hopkins_healthcare/downloads/cage%20substance %20screening%20tool.pdf. Accessed January 7, 2019.

21. Jahangard L, Akbarian S, Haghini M, et al. Children with ADHD and symptoms of oppositional defiant disorder improved in behavior when treated with methylphe-nidate and adjuvant risperidone, though weight gain was observed-results from a

randomized, double-blind, placebo controlled clinical trial. Psychiatry Res 2017. https://doi.org/10.1016/j.psychres.2016.12.010.

22. Wajszilber D, Santisiban JA, Gruber R. Sleep disorders in patients with ADHD: impact and management challenges. Nat Sci Sleep 2018. https://doi.org/10. 2147/NSS.S163074.

23. Tusaie K, Fitzpatrick JJ. Advanced practice psychiatric nursing, Second edition: Integrating psychotherapy, psychopharmacology and complementary approaches edited by Tusaie K, Fitzpatrick JJ. p. 430–1. Available at: https:// books.google.com/books?id=Wj0eDAAAQBAJ&pg=PA430&lpg=PA430&dq= Baseline+EKG+in+stimulant+induction&source=bl&ots=ifphqYAxbg&sig=946 lisJOqtzhmt7Qgo9z_cP_N9g&hl=en&sa=X&ved=2ahUKEwiQ8oetpd_fAhUjGz QIHah_AIUQ6AEwC3oECAMQAQ#v=onepage&q=Baseline%20EKG%20in%20 stimulant%20induction&f=false. Accessed January 8, 2019.

24. MGH. Psychiatric disorders during pregnancy, weighing the risks and benefits of pharmacologic treatment during pregnancy. Boston (MA): Massachusetts General Hospital Center for Women's Mental Health Reproductive Psychiatry Resource & Information Center; 2018. Webpage. Available at: https://womensmentalhealth. org/specialty-clinics/psychiatric-disorders-during-pregnancy/.

25. Americans with Disabilities Act 1990, with changes incorporated 2008. Webpage. Available at: https://www.ada.gov/pubs/ada.htm. Accessed January 4, 2018.

26. The National Institute of Mental Health (NIMH). Mental Health Information Hot Topics Attention Deficit-Hyperactivity Disorder. 2016. Available at: https://www.nimh.nih. gov/health/topics/attention-deficit-hyperactivity-disorder-adhd/index.shtml. Accessed January 8, 2019.

27. Committee on the Science of Changing Behavioral Health Social Norms, Board on Behavioral, Cognitive, and Sensory Sciences, Division of Behavioral and Social Sciences and Education, National Academies of Sciences, Engineering, and Medicine. 4, Approaches to Reducing Stigma. In: Ending discrimination against people with mental and substance use disorders: the evidence for stigma change. Washington (DC): National Academies Press (US); 2016. Available at: https://www.ncbi.nlm.nih.gov/books/NBK384914/. Accessed January 7, 2019.

28. NICHQ, American Academy of Pediatrics. NICHQ Vanderbilt assessment scales used for diagnosing ADHD. Available at: https://www.nichq.org/sites/default/files/ resource-file/NICHQ_Vanderbilt_Assessment_Scales.pdf. Accessed January 7, 2019.

29. Birmaher B, Brent DA, Chiappetta L, et al. Psychometric properties of the Screen for Child Anxiety Related Emotional Disorders (SCARED): a replication study. J Am Acad Child Adolesc Psychiatry 1999;38(10):1230–6.

30. Birmaher B. The Screen for Child Anxiety Related Disorders (SCARED). 1996. Available at: http://www.midss.org/content/screen-child-anxiety-related-disorders-scared. Accessed January 8, 2019.

31. Arab A, El Keshky M, Hadwin JA. Psychometric Properties of the Screen for Child Anxiety Related Emotional Disorders (SCARED) in a Non-Clinical Sample of Children and Adolescents in Saudi Arabia. Child Psychiatry Hum Dev 2015;47(4): 554–62. Available at: https://www.ncbi.nlm.nih.gov/pmc/articles/PMC4923097/. Accessed January 8, 2019.

32. Bright Futures. Tools for Professionals, Instructions for use. Pediatric Symptom Checklist for ages 4-17. Available at: https://www.brightfutures.org/mentalhealth/ pdf/professionals/ped_sympton_chklst.pdf. Accessed January 7, 2019.

33. Pappas D. ADHD rating scale-IV: checklists, norms, and clinical interpretation. J Psychoeduc Assess 2006;24(2):172–8.
34. CDC. My child has been diagnosed with ADHD-now what? Webpage. 2018. Available at: https://www.cdc.gov/ncbddd/adhd/treatment.html.
35. Clemow DB, Walker DJ. The potential for misuse and abuse of medications in ADHD: a review. Postgrad Med 2014;126(5):64–81.
36. Chang Z, Quinn PD, Hur K, et al. Association between medication use for attention-deficit/hyperactivity disorder and risk of motor vehicle crashes. JAMA Psychiatry 2017;74(6):597–603.
37. Bonham A. Why are 50 percent of pregnancies in the U.S. Unplanned? Special edition, a woman's nation changes everything. The Shriver Report 2018. Available at: http://shriverreport.org/why-are-50-percent-of-pregnancies-in-the-us-unplanned-adrienne-d-bonham/. Accessed November 15, 2018.
38. Transforming the understanding of mental illnesses. Attention-deficit/ hyperactivity disorder. National Institute of Mental Health. Webpage. Available at: https://www.nimh.nih.gov/health/topics/attention-deficit-hyperactivity-disorder-adhd/index.shtml. Accessed January 8 2019.
39. United States Food & Drug Administration. Dealing with ADHD: what you need to know. Rockville (MD): FDA; 2017. Available at: https://www.fda.gov/ForConsumers/ConsumerUpdates/ucm269188.htm. Accessed January 8, 2019.
40. Kooij JJ, Michielsen M, Kruithof H, et al. ADHD in old age: a review of the literature and proposal for assessment and treatment. Expert Rev Neurother 2016;16(12):1371–81.
41. Hennissen L, Bakker MJ, Banaschewski T, et al. Cardiovascular effects of stimulant and non-stimulant medication for children and adolescents with ADHD: a systematic review and meta-analysis of trials of methylphenidate, amphetamines and atomoxetine. CNS Drugs 2017;31:199–215.
42. Inglis SK, Carucci S, Garas P, et al, the ADDUCE Consortium. Prospective observational study protocol to investigate long-term adverse effects of methylphenidate in children and adolescents with ADHD: the Attention Deficit Hyperactivity Disorder Drugs Use Chronic Effects (ADDUCE) study. BMJ Open 2016;6:e010433.
43. Berger KH, Dillon KR, Sikkink KM, et al. Diversion of drugs within health care facilities, a multiple-victim crime: patterns of diversion, scope, consequences, detection, and prevention. Mayo Clin Proc 2012;87(7):674–82.
44. Ibrahim K, Donyai P. What stops practitioners discussing medication breaks in children and adolescents with ADHD? Identifying barriers through theory-driven qualitative research. Atten Defic Hyperact Disord 2018;10(4):273–83.
45. Barnard-Brak L, Roberts B, Valenzuela E. Examining breaks and resistance in medication adherence among adolescents with ADHD as associated with school outcomes. J Atten Disord 2018. https://doi.org/10.1177/1087054718763738.
46. Jensen ME, Pease EA, Lambert K, et al. Championing person-first language: a call to psychiatric mental health nurses. J Am Psychiatr Nurses Assoc 2013;19(3):146–51.
47. Jones T, Burhite B. Mental Health Stigma Reduction, Piloting the LINKS Anti-stigma Program. Poster. American Psychiatric Nurses Association Annual Conference, Indianapolis, IN. Available at: http://www.eventscribe.com/2018/posters/APNA/SplitViewer.asp?PID=MjgwODc3NDg4MzY. Accessed January 7, 2019.

48. Adams SM, Rice MJ, Jones SL, et al. TeleMental health: standards, reimbursement and interstate practice. J Am Psychiatr Nurses Assoc 2018;24(4): 295–305.

49. Harding KJK, Rush AJ, Arbuckle M, et al. Measurement-based care in psychiatric practice: a policy framework for implementation. J Clin Psychiatry 2011;72(8): 1136–43.

50. Hirsch JA, Rosenkrantz AB, Ansari SA, et al. MACRA 2.0: are you ready for MIPS? J Neurointerv Surg 2017;9:714–6. Available at: https://jnis-bmj-com.libproxy. usouthal.edu/content/9/7/714. Accessed November 25.

# Concordant Actions in Suicide Assessment Model

Sean P. Convoy, DNP, PMHNP-BC[a],*, Richard J. Westphal, PhD, PMHNP-BC, PMHCNS-BC[b,1],
Dana W. Convoy, BSN, RN-C[c,2]

## KEYWORDS

• Concordance • Locus of control • Suicide assessment • Suicide

## KEY POINTS

- Under optimal circumstances, health care providers can only influence, not control, patient suicide.
- Concordant actions in response to suicidal ideation and behavior accurately reflects health care provider's limited locus of control.
- Understanding the dynamics regarding locus of control is important for clinicians who are conducting suicide assessment.

## INTRODUCTION

According to the Centers for Disease Control (CDC), suicide is the 10th leading cause of death in the United States, exceeding 1.4 million attempts and 47,000 completions annually. If comparable national statistics reflected other medical conditions such as community-acquired pneumonia, Ebola, or H5N1, the CDC would have long since declared suicide a public health emergency. Notwithstanding the CDC's classification, suicide assessment is the responsibility of all nurses. The revised National Patient Safety Goals for 2019 require both an environmental and clinical risk assessment for suicide in all Joint Commission Accredited hospitals and behavioral health organizations.[1] Specifically, nurses and health care organizations will need to identify patients at risk and determine the severity of that risk to implement risk-reduction strategies.[2] Evidenced-based resources are available to support screening and assessment across a range of clinical settings and patient populations.[3] By design and necessity,

Disclosure: None of the authors of the article have research support, holds stock in, serves on an advisory board for any entity that would represent a conflict of interest related to this publication.
[a] Duke University School of Nursing, Durham, NC, USA; [b] University of Virginia at Charlottesville, P.O. Box 800782, McLeod Hall, Charlottesville, VA, USA; [c] United States Navy Reserve, Naval Operation Support Center, 3617 Carolina Beach Road, Wilmington, NC 28412, USA
[1] Present address: 137 Appalachian Lane, Gordonsville, VA 23942.
[2] Present address: 2900 Mills Lake Wynd, Holly Springs, NC 27540.
* Corresponding author. 2900 Mills Lake Wynd, Holly Springs, NC 27540.
E-mail address: sean.convoy@duke.edu

the screening tools assess suicide risk but not the severity or immediacy of suicide risk. To determine the severity or immediacy of suicide risk, the health care professional should perform an additional suicide safety assessment. An effective suicide safety assessment requires the clinician to establish a level of trust with the patient. A suicide safety assessment creates tension between the clinician and client. The clinician is obliged to conduct the assessment to predict the likelihood of self-harm action and to err on the side of safety when in doubt. Even if the client responds "no" to thoughts of suicide, it does not mean that he or she is safe. The client may be acutely aware that the assessment can lead to involuntary admission to a hospital or psychiatric facility. Understanding the dynamics regarding locus of control is important for clinicians who are conducting the suicide assessment. If they establish a relationship with patients, they are more likely to get truthful responses to their questions and make better decisions about patient safety.

## LOCUS OF CONTROL

To work effectively with clients who have suicidal thoughts and behavior, it is critical to step outside the clinic setting at times and meet the client where he or she is. All too often, a client report of suicidal thoughts in the clinical practice setting stimulates a rescue mentality in those who care for him or her.[4] While the notion of wanting to rescue someone before he harms himself is understandable, clinicians need to consider the impact of the loss of control an involuntary commitment could have on the patient over the long term. It is often negative.

One way to conceptualize suicidal thoughts and behavior is through the lens of locus of control. For some, suicidal thoughts and behaviors reflect the ultimate manifestation of control. Clients struggling with such thoughts may not be able to control or meaningfully influence their symptoms, stressors, or functioning in the present, but they can control when and if they take their own lives. Ironically, in an attempt to balance a patient's autonomy with a clinician's nonmaleficence, the clinician challenges a patient's control through involuntary or "coerced" hospitalization. Arguably, this action is justified by the clinician's interpretation of aggregate patient risk factors, inadequate exploration of health care professionals' countertransference, and unchecked concern about legal liability.[5,6] In essence, hospitalization becomes the clinician's path of least resistance. Clinician intrusion into a client's decision about suicide can unwittingly challenge locus of control and lead to a more permanent invocation of it. Those who struggle with suicidal thoughts and behaviors, as well as their caregivers, often focus on elements of the situation they cannot control while neglecting those they can.

The specter of suicide in clinical practice alters the perceptions of both the client and the clinician. To effectively work with suicidal patients, clinicians need to embrace a hard truth, which is that they have no control over outcomes. At best and under the right set of circumstances, clinicians can influence, but not control, outcomes. Assuming control of an individual's choice to take his or her life portends problems with clinician stress, burnout, and injury.[7,8]

## THEORETIC FRAME OF REFERENCE

After accepting the hard truth that clinical decisions cannot guarantee successful outcomes for suicidal patients, a different strategy surfaces. This strategy is informed by the collective works of Carl Rogers,[9,10] Hildegard Peplau,[11] and Kay Redfield Jamison.[12,13]

Rogers' person-centered approach to psychology is defined by 3 pillars: congruence (authenticity and genuineness), accurate empathy, and unconditional positive regard (nonjudgmental stance).[9] He identifies 6 necessary and sufficient conditions for therapeutic personality change, 7 stages of process that refer to how change manifests over time, and 19 propositions that describe the nature of human personality and how it works. Roger's humanistic approach recognizes that any attempt to influence a client's thoughts about suicide must begin with mutual trust and respect—even around an individual's decisions about suicide. Roger's person-centered approach allows the clinician to see the tree through the forest and encourages him or her to put more effort into the therapeutic relationship and less into controlling a client's behavior. Once a clinician accepts the premise that he or she has no real control (except when patients do not demonstrate a capacity for decision making), demonstrating *unconditional positive regard* is the only purposeful action to take under such circumstances.

Peplau's Theory of Interpersonal Relationships defines purposeful interaction between 2 or more individuals who communicate, transfer values, and produce energy from within their unique roles in society.[14] Her 6 nursing roles (eg, *stranger*, *resource*, *teaching*, *counseling*, *surrogate*, and *leadership*) as well as developmental stages of the nurse-client relationship (eg, *orientation*, *identification*, *exploitation*, and *resolution*) are internally consistent with Rogerian theory in that they see the therapeutic relationship as more a product of support, acceptance, and influence than control. Peplau's work operationalizes a process to develop rapport, trust, and problem solving through the therapeutic use of self. Again, accepting the premise that the clinician has no real control, leveraging the therapeutic relationship is the only purposeful action to take.

Jamison's exhaustive efforts focus on deconstructing suicide and destigmatizing mental illness through the juxtaposition of scientific evidence and anecdotal stories, making the complex suicidal condition easier to comprehend. She argues that suicide commonly coexists alongside mental illness and any attempt to treat or manage one without adequate consideration of the other is a fool's errand. Jamison contends that the US mental health care delivery systems' approach to suicide is tantamount to a team's defending the football on its own 2-yard line. Earlier in the game, plays on the field are important in preventing a goal-line defense. In mental health care, strategies proximal to the cause of the diagnosis can have a profound influence on patient outcomes. Jamison advises clinicians to spend less time trying to control the phenomenon of suicide and more time trying to understand the individual and the meaning behind suicide in his or her life.

The work of Rogers, Peplau, and Jamison provided the kindling for the concept of Concordant Actions in Suicide Assessment (CASA), a model designed to help clinicians see and respond to the phenomenon of suicide differently.

## CONCORDANT ACTIONS IN SUICIDE ASSESSMENT MODEL

The CASA model establishes 3 steps in the process of caring for a patient with suicidal thoughts and/or behavior: *suicidal symptom recognition*, *clinician decision*, and the *suicide continuum*.

Not all aspects of suicidal thinking and behavior are observable. The subjective elements of suicide both precede and significantly outweigh the objective signs of suicidal thoughts and behaviors. For many individuals, the struggle with suicide is years and even decades long. Generally, the health care delivery system only responds to suicidal thoughts and behaviors when patients in trouble cross clinical thresholds. Those clinical thresholds also vary tremendously across the health care delivery system. Far too many variables make it impossible to meaningfully predict, let alone control, individual outcomes. For the purposes of this model, *suicidal symptom recognition* is defined as the point at which a clinician is aware of suicide's presence in a client's life.

The second step in the process is *clinician decision*. After a clinician recognizes suicidal symptoms, he or she has decisions to make and actions to take. Variables that influence a clinician's decision making include his or her formal education, clinical practice experience, institutional guidance, countertransference, and moral distress and residue,[15,16] as well as the provider's own relative health. The provider then has 2 approaches. He or she can be informed by aggregate risk factors, societal laws, practice guidelines, herd mentality, and risk aversion (state action). Or the provider can act through the prism of concordance and be informed by the client's truth, power, authority, and potential opportunities for growth.

The third element of the model establishes the *suicide continuum* that ranges from fleeting thoughts of nonexistence to suicidal behavior. Individuals exist somewhere along this continuum at any given time. The line of suicidal symptom recognition bisects the continuum.

Evidence-informed models may be useful heuristic representations of dynamic or complex relations and concepts. The CASA model is a graphic representation of a clinician's assessment in the context of a client's continuum of suicidal thoughts and behaviors (**Fig. 1**). The model begins with the need to assess suicidal risk. The results of a suicide screen or a client's symptoms trigger the assessment. The second element in the model is the clinician's preparation for engaging and assessing the client. In this step, the clinician must blend therapeutic alliance and trust building with regulatory and organizational standards on patient safety to create a treatment plan. The third step recognizes that suicidal thinking occurs along a continuum ranging from fleeting thoughts of nonexistence through the intent to end one's life. The CASA model highlights a concordant approach in which clinicians recognize, acknowledge, and use strategies to reduce the risk that a patient will act on suicidal thoughts. Conversely, when clinicians principally focus on suicidal ideation and behavior, they may miss opportunities to support client self-agency and less restrictive means to support safety.

## APPLICATION OF THE MODEL

A clinical exemplar offers an illustration of how the CASA may be useful in the clinical setting.

## Concordant Actions in Suicide Assessment Model

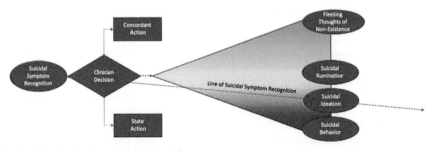

**Fig. 1.** Suicide decision-making model.

As the clinical exemplar establishes (**Box 1**), Aiden has struggled with suicidal ideations for the better part of a decade. However, it was only after the clinician used the Columbia-Suicide Severity Rating Scale[17] that Aiden's suicidal symptoms were recognized as a clinical priority. After recognizing the symptoms, the clinician has decisions to make and actions to take. The clinician could rely on his or her formal education and training, which often frames suicide as a "permanent solution to a temporary problem." The clinician could spend time exploring Aiden's risk factors for suicide or looking for clinical practice guidelines that attempt to quantify the relative risk and to guide care in a presumed evidence-based direction. The clinician could explore Aiden's safety history; evidence suggests past suicidal behavior is a good predictor of future behavior. In the absence of a declarative assertion that Aiden is not at immediate risk for suicide, the clinician could reasonably err on the side of caution and pursue psychiatric hospitalization. Such actions would not necessarily be wrong. However, in the absence a substantive exploration of Aiden as an individual, they would arguably reflect a *state action*.

Alternatively, the clinician could approach Aiden's symptoms from a different perspective. Informed by the work of Rogers, Peplau, and Jamison, the clinician could spend time getting to know Aiden. He or she could explore what meaning and purpose suicide serves in Aiden's life. The clinician could investigate how Aiden's chronic depression and trauma-based symptoms inform his suicidal symptoms. The clinician could candidly declare the inability to control Aiden's choice but passionately invoke the desire to assist him in better managing his symptoms. The clinician could assert Aiden's control and reframe his suicidal ideations as a reasonable response to an unmet need. See **Box 2** for an example of these concordant action.

As can be seen in the exemplar, the concordant action fully acknowledges and embraces the client's locus of control. There are no overt attempts to subvert the client's will. Rather, the approach merely attempts to place alternatives between a patient's present reality and suicide. The approach merely attempts to shift the risk to the right, which might seem inadequate given the potentially lethal outcome. However, returning to the premise that the provider has no meaningful control over the outcome, this approach is a pragmatic position that invests more time and effort into the therapeutic relationship (*that which we can control*) than the ultimate decision associated with suicide (*that which we cannot control*).

The application of a cognitive reframe informed by concordance will not resolve suicidal symptoms for patients actively struggling with psychosis, mania, neurocognitive symptoms, or acute substance intoxication. This approach is not necessarily an alternative to purposeful state actions, but rather an augmented approach that might help the client manage suicidal thoughts and behaviors.

---

**Box 1**
**Clinical exemplar, part 1**

Aiden is a recently separated military veteran with an extensive mental health history that, to some degree, informs his service release. Aiden has since established his health care with the Department of Veteran Affairs (VA). Aiden has struggled with suicidal ideations for more than a decade with a history of 2 past attempts during his active-duty service time, both informed by acute substance intoxication. Aiden presents to his first VA mental health appointment for management of chronic mood- and trauma-based symptoms. During the initial screening process, Aiden completed the Columbia-Suicide Severity Rating Scale, which sensitized the clinician to Aiden's active suicidal ideations. On recognition of suicidal symptoms, the clinician appropriately shifted clinical focus from the chronic mood- and trauma-based symptoms to the active suicidal ideations.

**Box 2**
**Clinical exemplar, part 2, the concordant action**

Clinician: "I see by the screening tool you filled out that you're struggling with suicidal thoughts."

Client: "Yes, that is not anything new in my life."

Clinician: "Can we agree that if you want to take your life there is not much I can actually do prevent you?"

Client: "You may be able to slow me down but not really stop me."

Clinician: "I appreciate that observation. So, while I might be able to temporarily prevent you from taking your life, I can't permanently prevent you from taking your life. Is that correct?"

Client: "Yeah. If I'm going to do it, I'm going to do it."

Clinician: "So, you are in complete control of this. You could choose to do it today, tomorrow, six years from now, or never. Is that right?"

Client: "Again, yes. You sure do like to talk about this stuff."

Clinician: "I'm funny that way. OK, let me shift focus for a minute. Do you think it reasonable to suggest you have tried every possible strategy to get better?"

Client: "I've tried a lot of things but if I am going to be honest about it, I don't think I have tried everything."

Clinician: "Again, I appreciate your objectivity. All considered, since you essentially control when and if you are going to take your life and you haven't really tried all possible options to get better, what would be the harm of giving yourself some more time before you make such a big decision? I'm not asking you for a safety contract that says you will never kill yourself. That stuff doesn't work. I am asking for an opportunity to help you try some more things before you make that big decision."

Client: "Every time someone has talked with me about suicide in the past they try to pin me down about it. It's kind of weird that you, the mental health professional, are not taking suicide off the table."

Clinician: "Again, I'm funny that way. How can I take something off the table that I am unable to control? Let me shift focus again. I would like to spend some time getting to better understand you. I believe suicidal thoughts can be in response to unmet needs. I'd like to better understand how these thoughts work in your life."

Client: "OK, how do you want to start?"

## RECOGNITION

The CASA model is the culmination of 20 years of study and clinical experience while serving in the United States Navy and Marine Corps. The military's mental health care delivery system has been forced to drink responsibly from the fire hose of crisis intervention for far too long, with the unreasonable expectation that its health care professionals should predict and prevent suicide, personally own missed opportunities to do so, and privately navigate the sequela.

## ACKNOWLEDGMENTS

The authors are grateful to Carl Rogers, Ph.D., Hildegard Peplau, Ed.D, and Kay Redfield Jamison, Ph.D., for significantly informing this work. Specifically, Dr Jamison's books, *An Unquiet Mind*[12] and *Night Falls Fast: Understanding Suicide*,[13] have been transformative in our understanding of the subject.

## REFERENCES

1. The Joint Commission. Joint commission announces newnational patient safety goal to prevent suicide and improve at-risk patient care. The Joint Commission; 2018. Available at: https://www.jointcommission.org/joint_commission_announces_new_national_patient_safety_goal_to_prevent_suicide_and_improve_at-risk_patient_care/.
2. The Joint Commission. National Patient Safety Goal (NPSG) Effective January 2019. The Joint Commission; 2019. Available at: https://www.jointcommission.org/assets/1/6/NPSG_Chapter_HAP_Jan2019.pdf.
3. The Joint Commission. Suicide prevention resources to support Joint Commission accredited organizations implementation of NPSG 15.01.01. The Joint Commission; 2019. Available at: https://www.jointcommission.org/npsg_150101_suicide_prevention_resources/.
4. Wang DWL, Colucci E. Should compulsory admission to hospital be part of suicide prevention strategies? BJPsych Bull 2017;41(3):169–71.
5. Berge T, Bjøntegård KS, Ekern P, et al. Coercive mental health care — dilemmas in the decision-making process. Tidsskr Nor Laegeforen 2018;138(12).
6. Yaseen ZS, Briggs J, Kopeykina I, et al. Distinctive emotional responses of clinicians to suicide-attempting patients — a comparative study. BMC Psychiatry 2013;13:230.
7. Draper B, Kõlves K, De Leo D, et al. The impact of patient suicide and sudden death on health care professionals. Gen Hosp Psychiatry 2014;36(6):721–5.
8. Oravecz R, Moore MM. Recognition of suicide risk according to the characteristics of the suicide process. Death Stud 2006;30(3):269–79.
9. Rogers CR. Client-centered therapy, its current practice, implications, and theory. The Houghton Mifflin psychological series. Boston: Houghton Mifflin; 1951. p. 560, xii.
10. Rogers CR, American Psychological Association. Client-centered therapy. Washington, DC: American Psychological Association; 1985.
11. Peplau HE. Peplau's theory of interpersonal relations. Nurs Sci Q 1997;10(4):162–7.
12. Jamison KR. An unquiet mind. 1st edition. New York: A.A. Knopf; 1995. p. 223.
13. Jamison KR. Night falls fast: understanding suicide. 1st edition. New York: Knopf; 1999. p. 432.
14. Peplau HE. Interpersonal techniques: the crux of psychiatric nursing. Am J Nurs 1962;62:50–4.
15. Hamric AB. Moral distress in everyday ethics. Nurs Outlook 2000;48(5):199–201.
16. Hamric AB, Davis WS, Childress MD. Moral distress in health care professionals. Pharos Alpha Omega Alpha Honor Med Soc 2006;69(1):16–23.
17. Matarazzo BB, Brown GK, Stanley B, et al. Predictive validity of the Columbia-Suicide Severity Rating Scale among a cohort of at-risk veterans. Suicide Life Threat Behav 2018. https://doi.org/10.1111/sltb.12515.

# Delirium Superimposed on Dementia

## Challenges and Opportunities

Evelyn Parrish, PhD, PMHNP-BC

## KEYWORDS

- Delirium • Dementia • Delirium superimposed on dementia • Treatment

## KEY POINTS

- Delirium is an acute medical emergency that is not easily detected, and is typically caused by a systemic infection, medication related, or an underlying illness.
- The symptoms of delirium and dementia are similar, which contributes to the difficulty in detecting delirium.
- Nurses and nursing staff are key to early detection of symptoms of delirium.
- Nurses and nursing staff need the proper training and education in the area of assessment for symptoms of delirium.

## INTRODUCTION

Numerous medical advances have occurred during the past decade that have contributed to people living longer. At present in the United States, those 65 years of age and older comprise approximately 16% of the total population and it is expected that by 2030 they will make up approximately 21% of the population.[1] According to the World Health Organization,[2] common illnesses that occur in older age include hypertension, diabetes, depression, dementia, hearing loss, vision loss, back pain, chronic obstructive pulmonary disease, and osteoarthritis. The demands for and on health care services are likely to increase at a more rapid rate than has been seen in the past.

This age group is also more likely to have comorbid or multimorbid conditions that can lead to an increased rate of functional decline.[3] Persons with multiple chronic conditions require frequent health care provider visits, hospitalizations, in-home services, long-term care, and more medications.[4] In addition, many illnesses share the same or similar symptoms, making it difficult to determine the appropriate treatment regimen. The aging of America presents clinicians with many opportunities to address, and these are beyond the scope of this article.

Disclosure: The author has no disclosures to report.
University of Kentucky College of Nursing, 202 College of Nursing Building, Lexington, KY 40536, USA
E-mail address: Evelyn.parrish@uky.edu

This article discusses the identification of symptoms and treatment options for patients who experience delirium superimposed on dementia.

## BACKGROUND

Delirium and dementia are cognitive syndromes common in the elderly population. Delirium is an acute, common, and serious medical condition characterized by a rapid onset with a decline in level of cognition and concurrent fluctuations in mood, perception, and behavior.[5] Delirium occurs in up to 25% of hospitalized patients, 20% in nursing home patients, 50% in postsurgery patients, 75% in intensive care unit (ICU) patients, and 50% in patients with dementia.[6,7] Delirium can occur in any age group but is slightly more common in people less than 3 and more than 70 years of age.[8] Delirium is associated with adverse outcomes, which include increased mortality, increased falls, functional decline, and cognitive impairment. In 2011, the direct and indirect costs for the treatment of delirium were $152 billion per year.[8,9]

Dementia was termed a neurocognitive disorder in the Diagnostic and Statistical Manual of Mental Disorders, Fifth Edition (DSM-5)[5] and is a chronic, progressive cluster of symptoms that causes decline in cognitive functioning and worsens over time. The World Health Organization[2] reported that in 2017 approximately 50 million people were diagnosed with dementia and that it was the seventh leading cause of death. Because it is a progressive disease, the impact on the individual and family are gradual. As the disease progresses the greatest impact is on the family and caregivers as the patient requires more care. The costs of health care and long-term care for individuals with Alzheimer or other dementias are substantial, and dementia is one of the costliest conditions to society. In 2018, the cost of care for all individuals with Alzheimer or other dementias was approximately $277 billion and by 2050 it is estimated to be approximately $1.1 trillion.[10]

Delirium superimposed on dementia is often undiagnosed or misdiagnosed as the worsening of the symptoms of dementia or depression.[11,12] Reynish and colleagues[13] reported that patients with delirium superimposed on dementia have longer hospital stays and increased mortality 30 days from admission and 1 year from admission compared with patients diagnosed with delirium. Patients with dementia experienced a higher rate of mortality 1 year from admission than patients with delirium superimposed on dementia.[13]

## DISCUSSION
### Pathophysiology

Although the pathophysiology of delirium is not well understood, Maldonado[14] proposes that, "the specific combination of neurotransmitter dysfunction and the variability in integration and appropriate processing of sensory information and motor responses, as well as the degree of breakdown in cerebral network connectivity directly, contribute to the various cognitive and behavioral changes, as well as the clinical motoric phenotype observed in delirium." In addition, there are 2 types of delirium: hypoactive and hyperactive. Hölttäcolleagues[15] reported that hypoactive delirium was more common in patients with delirium and with dementia.

Dementia is a symptom of a variety of specific structural brain diseases and degenerative processes. Several diseases can cause dementia, including Alzheimer, vascular dementia, Lewy body dementia, Parkinson disease, frontotemporal dementia, Creutzfeldt-Jakob disease, Wernicke-Korsakoff syndrome, and Huntington disease.[5] Each have specific causes and symptoms based on the area of the brain that is affected.

Delirium and dementia have common pathophysiologic and clinical presentation characteristics. These characteristics include decreased cholinergic neurotransmission and increased systemic and neural inflammation[12] that lead to increased cognitive decline. They share some commonalities in pathology and symptoms as well as differences, which contribute to the difficulty of recognizing and treating the delirium early, especially when it occurs in patients with dementia.

### Precipitating and Risk Factors of Delirium

Several factors have been identified that often precipitate patients experiencing symptoms of delirium. These factors include medications, such as sedatives, narcotics, anticholinergics, polypharmacy, and alcohol withdrawal; having a primary neurologic disease; surgical procedures; and environmental issues, such as being admitted to an ICU, placed in physical restraints, bladder catheter, multiple procedures in a short period of time, physical pain, and emotional distress.[14,15] Several risk factors can increase the likelihood of developing delirium, including being 65 years of age and older; being female; dementia; history of delirium; depression; decreased mobility; increased dependence; history of falls; dehydration; malnutrition; fecal impaction; sensory impairments; psychotropic medications; polypharmacy; alcohol abuse; respiratory infections; urinary tract infections; dehydration; malnutrition; fecal impaction; chronic pain; and urinary retention.[14–18] Many people 65 years of age and older have or will have some of these precipitating and risk factors requiring more astute and knowledgeable health care providers in the management of both delirium and dementia.

### Symptoms

The symptom presentations of delirium and dementia are similar as well as different. To accurately assess patients with delirium, most health care providers could benefit from a review. Delirium has 2 subtypes: hypoactive and hyperactive.[19] The symptom presentation of each subtype is reflective of the name; for example, in hypoactive delirium the symptoms include drowsiness, decreased alertness, and withdrawn. Patients with hyperactive delirium show agitation, irritability, decreased sleep, and hypervigilance. The clinical symptoms of both subtypes of delirium are presented in **Table 1**.[11,17,19]

The key to understanding and recognizing the symptoms of delirium and dementia, especially delirium superimposed on dementia, is in their differences. Although all features are considered, confusion and disorientation are considered the hallmark symptoms for both delirium and dementia, taking into consideration the rate of onset. The level of confusion and orientation in a patient with dementia takes months to change, but hours to days in delirium. A comparison of the features of delirium and dementia is presented in **Table 2**.[6,12,16–21]

### Assessment

The assessment of delirium, especially when superimposed on dementia, is difficult at best because of the similarities in the pathology and symptom presentation. The use of a comprehensive and holistic assessment is the best approach to take in determining what is going on with the patient. Frequently, patients with dementia are either being cared for in the home of a relative or in a long-term care facility. Regardless of their place of residence, the assessment must include collateral information from the identified caregiver/family member. Some key questions to ask the caregiver/family include what the patient's behavior was before this event/illness; what the patient's behavior is usually like; and whether the patient has ever been like this before (if yes, when, and describe the event/illness). Engage the caregiver/family in all aspects

**Table 1**
**Symptom presentation in delirium**

| Clinical Feature | Hypoactive Delirium | Hyperactive Delirium |
|---|---|---|
| Arousal | Decreased arousal; decreased alertness; drowsiness; reduced awareness of surroundings | Hypervigilant; distractible; startles easily |
| Onset | Abrupt onset; fluctuating course | Abrupt onset; fluctuating course |
| Perceptual disturbance | Visual hallucinations; misperceptions; illusions | Visual hallucinations; misperceptions; illusions |
| Disturbance of thought content | Paranoid delusions: vague and not systematic | Persistent thoughts and delusions are more common |
| Mood symptoms | Sad; depressed; irritable; labile; disinhibited | Mood lability: may include a wide range of mood states from combative or impatient to euphoric |
| Psychomotor activity | Slowed down; withdrawn; quiet | Restless; agitated |
| Past psychiatric history | May have a history of delirium | Correlated with alcohol and/or drug withdrawal; may have a history of delirium |
| Sleep-wake disturbance | Increased daytime sleepiness | Prominent sleep-wake disturbance- nightmares/night terrors |

*Data from* Refs.[11,17,19]

**Table 2**
**Comparison of delirium and dementia features**

| Feature | Delirium | Dementia |
|---|---|---|
| Onset | Sudden and abrupt depending on cause; occurs most often at dusk | Insidious, slow, and often unrecognized during the early stages |
| Course | Depends on timely diagnosis and treatment; can be short and reversible | Progressive; currently only pharmacologic agents to slow the progression |
| Duration | Short: hours to days; longer in some if unrecognized and/or untreated | Terminal illness: months to years |
| Orientation | Generally impaired initially; disoriented to time and place; usually regains after effectively treated | Level of impairment varies depending on stage of illness |
| Memory | Generally impaired initially; unable to recall events of hospitalization/illness, or follow instructions; usually regains after effectively treated | Initially loses short-term memory and as disease progresses so does the degree of memory loss |
| Psychomotor | Hypoactive: increased drowsiness and daytime sedation. Hyperactive: decreased sleep, agitated and restless; hallucinations and delusions may occur if undiagnosed/untreated | Level of impairment depends on the stage: restless, agitated, afraid, hallucinations, and delusions as the disease progresses |

*Data from* Refs.[6,12,16–21]

of the patient's care especially if the patient is in a long-term care facility. Other items to assess include whether the symptoms wax and wane over a 24-hour period; whether the patient has fluctuations between lethargy and restlessness over several hours; whether the patient is attentive when addressed by someone; whether the patient makes eye contact; whether the patient makes sense when responding to questions; and whether the patient is experiencing lethargy/somnolence or restless/agitated behavior which is different from the baseline. Further assessment of symptoms of delirium and a comparison with those seen in patients with dementia are outlined in **Table 3**.

The assessment of the patient includes level of acuity of mental status change; review of the results of the assessment scales, such as the Confusion Assessment Method[22]; and whether the presentation is atypical (consider myocardial infarction, infection, respiratory failure). Obtain and review the following laboratory assessments, which assist in confirming a diagnosis: complete blood count with differential, blood cultures, chest radiograph, and urinalysis (rule out an infectious process); electrolytes, blood urea nitrogen, creatinine, glucose (rule out dehydration and electrolyte imbalances); blood and urine drug screens (rule out any drug toxicity); thyroid-stimulating hormone (rule out thyroid issues); calcium, albumin (rule out malnutrition); liver function (rule out hepatic issues); and Venereal Disease Research Laboratory test (rule out venereal disease).[6,20,21,23,24]

Another component of the patient assessment includes a review of the patient's current and immediate past medications. The medication regimen of patients with dementia typically includes multiple medications, which can often have interactions or side effects that could contribute to behavioral changes. As the patient's level of confusion/agitation increases, other mediations may be added. Medications that have anticholinergic side effects and can contribute to the development of delirium as well as cognitive and behavioral changes include some of the drugs in the following classes: benzodiazepines, diphenhydramine, antibiotics, antihypertensive,

**Table 3**
**Assessment of delirium**

|  | Delirium Indicator | Method of Assessment | Delirium vs Dementia |
|---|---|---|---|
| Acute onset | Symptoms develop within hours to days | Determine baseline before this event. Assess the ability to perform ADLs | Changes in dementia are slow, occurring over months to years |
| Fluctuating course | Symptoms wax and wane over a 24-h period | Assess if patient has periods of lucidness with confusion | In dementia, some behaviors may fluctuate |
| Inattention | Difficulty focusing | Assess level on concentration and ability to follow directions | In dementia, patients are able to focus during interactions with others until they are in the advanced stages |
| Disorganized thinking | Answers are rambling and speech maybe nonsensical | Assess understanding and responses | In dementia: in early stage, responses make sense |
| Altered level of alertness | Either decrease or increase in level of alertness | Assess level of behavior and alertness | Level of alertness is not altered in dementia |

*Abbreviation:* ADLs, activities of daily living.

antidepressants, antipsychotics, and anticoagulants. To determine the anticholinergic impact that patients' medications can have on their cognitive functioning, Boustani and colleagues[25] developed the Anticholinergic Burden Scale. The scale contains a list of medications that are divided by the degree to which they affect acetylcholine activity, from 1 (little cognitive effect) to 3 (clinically significant cognitive effect). The patient's medications are compared with those in the list and scored accordingly. A score of 3 or greater is an indication to change medications to one in the lower effect category. Another consideration with regard to medications is whether the patient is taking the medications as directed, which may not be an issue if the patient has been in a long-term care facility.

The total assessment of the patient is critical and should include the use of assessment tools to screen for both delirium and dementia. Some of the more common assessment tools that are well validated are included in **Table 4**. The Confusion Assessment Method[22] has been repeatedly used in the assessment of delirium and particularly in patients with dementia. The assessment may require multiple tools to fully evaluate the patient's level of dementia and delirium.

All of the diagnostic criteria as outlined in the DSM-5[5] have to be met to confirm the diagnosis of delirium, and include disturbance in attention and awareness; develops acutely and fluctuates in severity; 1 additional disturbance in cognition; not better explained by preexisting dementia; does not occur in a severely reduced level of arousal or coma; and evidence of an underlying organic cause.[5]

### Treatment

The prevention of delirium in patients with dementia is the primary goal. Some preventive measures include ensuring that the patient has adequate nutrition, hydration, and sleep; bowel regimen protocol; assessing for changes in level of cognitive functioning; avoiding benzodiazepines, diphenhydramine, and other anticholinergics; and ensuring that patients have their eyeglasses and/or hearing aids.[32,33] The treatment of delirium is as complicated as the diagnosing because of the fluctuations in symptom presentation, which may be the result of the delirium or the dementia. The primary goal is to

| Table 4 | |
|---|---|
| **Delirium and dementia assessment tools** | |
| **Measure** | **Purpose** |
| Delirium | |
| Confusion Assessment Method[25] | Identify delirium in clinical and research settings |
| 4AT Rapid Assessment Test[26] | Assess for delirium in routine, nonspecialist clinic visits |
| Richmond Agitation and Sedation Scale[27] | Measures agitation and sedation level |
| Dementia | |
| Montreal Cognitive Assessment[28] | Assess orientation, attention, memory, language, and visual construction |
| Dementia Rating Scale-2[29] | Measures cognitive functioning in adults with neurologic disturbance |
| Repeatable Battery for the Assessment of Neuropsychological Status[30] | Measures cognitive functioning in adults with neurologic disturbance |
| Mini-Mental State Examination[31] | Screen for mental impairment |

Abbreviations: 4AT, 4 item assessment test for delirium.
Data from Refs.[25–31]

reverse the symptoms to end any potentially dangerous behaviors. Both nonpharmacologic and pharmacologic treatment modalities should be considered. Nonpharmacologic management strategies include reorientation; explaining everything to the patient; sleep hygiene; making eyeglasses or other vision aids accessible to the patient; making hearing aids accessible to the patient; making hydrating liquids accessible to the patient; ensuring adequate nutrition (ask the family to bring in the patient's favorite food); avoiding restraints; making all interactions respectful and courteous; encouraging the family to be present when they are available; and communicating with family at a minimum of weekly with an update on the patient's condition.[32,33]

The pharmacologic treatment of delirium is focused on treating the underlying cause. The management of other symptoms also needs to be addressed. Second-generation antipsychotic agents have been used to treat the behavioral and psychological symptoms with mild to moderate benefit.[19,23,34] At present, all antipsychotic agents carry a black box warning regarding use in the elderly population, which requires an assessment of the risks and benefits of using the medication. It is important to remember the onset of action for the medications to gauge whether the medication was helpful in decreasing the behavior or not. Patients may receive medications for their behavioral symptoms and calm before the medication has reached its onset of action.

## SUMMARY

Patients who are 65 years of age and older and those with existing cognitive impairment have an increased risk of developing delirium. Delirium superimposed on dementia is a common and treatable illness if detected early. Delirium is difficult to detect and is more complicated when the patient has dementia.[13] A complete and holistic assessment including physical assessment, laboratory tests, review of medications and medical history, and assessment tools is essential in determining the underlying cause of the delirium.[14,15] Obtaining collateral information for the family and/or caregiver should be included in the assessment because this often has historical information about the patient.

The most effective treatment of delirium is the prevention of delirium. Preventive measures and nonpharmacologic supportive care measures should become the standard for all patients, especially with dementia, regardless of their living situations. The pharmacologic management of delirium is to alleviate the cause and control the behavioral and psychological symptoms.[14–17]

The management of patients with delirium superimposed on dementia is ongoing and requires frequent reassessment to monitor the level of delirium even when patients are symptom free. These patients are most often in a long-term care facility or palliative care center where they are cared for by nurses and nursing staff. Yevchak and colleagues[35] reported on the use of a nurse-facilitated person-centered care model that is the standard of care for patients with delirium superimposed on dementia. Each patient's intake should include the results of a physical examination, laboratory screens, medication history, psychosocial history, delirium and dementia assessment tool scores, and collateral information from the family to establish the patient's baseline information. Fick and colleagues[36] reported on the use of case vignettes to assess the nursing staffs' knowledge of their patients. Although the staff knew their patients, they did not have the necessary information and training to perform an assessment for delirium. Hasemann and colleagues[37] reported on the nurses' recognition of symptoms of delirium in patients with cognitive impairment using the Delirium Observation Screening Scale and the Confusion Assessment Method Scale. The nurses were able to identify symptoms of delirium, hyperactivity type, whereas they missed the symptoms of delirium, hypoactive type. With the necessary training and education, nurses and nursing staff are the key to the early detection of symptoms of delirium. Delirium is an acute medical emergency that is difficult to detect. Patients with delirium superimposed on dementia tend to have longer hospitalizations, frequent readmissions, and higher mortalities than others. Health care providers have to be aware of and identify the symptoms of delirium for the patients to have the best outcomes.

## REFERENCES

1. US Census Bureau. Available at: https://www.census.gov/library/stories/2018/03/graying-america.html. Accessed November 9, 2018.
2. World Health Organization. Available at: https://www.who.int/news-room/fact-sheets/detail/ageing-and-health. Accessed November 9, 2018.
3. Zulman D, Martins S, Liu Y, et al. Using a clinical knowledge base to assess co-morbidity interrelatedness among patients with multiple chronic conditions. AMIA Annu Symp Proc 2015;2015:1381–9.
4. Zulman DM, Asch SM, Martins SB, et al. Quality of care for patients with multiple chronic conditions: the role of comorbidity interrelatedness. J Gen Intern Med 2013;29(3):529–37.
5. American Psychiatric Association. Diagnostic and statistical manual of mental disorders: DSM-5. 5th edition. Arlington (VA): American Psychiatric Association; 2013.
6. Fong TG, Davis D, Growdon ME. The interface between delirium and dementia in elderly adults. Lancet Neurol 2015;14(8):823–32.
7. Delirium Organization. Available at: http://www.idelirium.org/about-delirium.html. Accessed December 20, 2018.
8. Inouye S, Westendorp R, Saczynski J. Delirium in elderly people. Lancet 2014; 383(9920):911–22.
9. Leslie DL, Inouye SK. The importance of Delirium: Economic and Societal costs. J Am Geriatr Soc 2011;59:S241–3.
10. Alzheimer's Organization-facts and figures. Available at: https://www.alz.org/media/Documents/alzheimers-facts-and-figures-infographic.pdf. Accessed December 1, 2018.
11. Apold S. Delirium superimposed on dementia. J Nurse Pract 2018;14(3):183–9.
12. Leonard A, Spiller D, Mohamad M, et al. Delirium diagnostic and classification challenges in palliative care: subsyndromal delirium, comorbid delirium-dementia, and psychomotor subtypes. J Pain Symptom Manage 2014;48(2):199–214.
13. Reynish E, Hapca S, Cvoro V, et al. Epidemiology and outcomes of people with dementia, delirium, and unspecified cognitive impairment in the general hospital: Prospective cohort study of 10,014 admissions. BMC Med 2017;15(1):1–12.
14. Maldonado J. Delirium pathophysiology: an updated hypothesis of the etiology of acute brain failure. Int J Geriatr Psychiatry 2018;33:1428–57.
15. Hölttä EH, Laurila JV, Laakkonen ML, et al. Precipitating factors of delirium: stress response to multiple triggers among patients with and without dementia. Exp Gerontol 2014;59:42–6.

16. Fong T, Albuquerque A, Inouye S. The search for effective delirium treatment for persons with dementia in the postacute-care setting. J Am Geriatr Soc 2016; 64(12):2421–3.
17. Brooke J. Differentiation of delirium, dementia and delirium superimposed on dementia in the older person. Br J Nurs 2018;27(7):363–7.
18. Fick DM, Steis MR, Waller JL, et al. Delirium superimposed on dementia is associated with prolonged length of stay and poor outcomes in hospitalized older adults. J Hosp Med 2013;8(9):500–5.
19. Downing L, Caprio J, Lyness T. Geriatric psychiatry review: differential diagnosis and treatment of the 3 D's - delirium, dementia, and depression. Curr Psychiatry Rep 2013;15(6):1–10.
20. Morandi A, Bellelli D, Caplan A, et al. The diagnosis of delirium superimposed on dementia: an emerging challenge. J Am Med Dir Assoc 2017;18(1):12–8.
21. Landreville P, Voyer P, Carmichael PH. Relationship between delirium and behavioral symptoms in dementia. Int Psychogeriatr 2013;25(4):635–43.
22. Inouye S, Van Dyck C, Alessi C, et al. Clarifying confusion: the confusion assessment method. A new method for detection of delirium. Ann Intern Med 1990; 113(12):941–8.
23. Hshieh T, Inouye S, Oh E. Delirium in the elderly. Psychiatr Clin North Am 2018; 41(1):1–17.
24. Jackson T, Gladman J, Harwood R, et al. Challenges and opportunities in understanding dementia and delirium in the acute hospital. PLoS Med 2017;14(3): E1002247.
25. Boustani M, Campbell N, Munger S, et al. Impact of anticholinergics on the aging brain: a review and practical application. Aging Health 2008;4(3):311–20.
26. 4AT assessment scale. Available at: https://www.the4at.com/. Accessed December 21, 2018.
27. Sessler CN, Gosnell MS, Grap MJ, et al. The Richmond agitation-sedation scale: validity and reliability in adult intensive care unit patients. Am J Respir Crit Care Med 2002;166(10):1338–44.
28. Nasreddine ZS, Phillips NA, Bédirian V, et al. The montreal cognitive assessment, MoCA: a brief screening tool for mild cognitive impairment. J Am Geriatr Soc 2005;53(4):695–9.
29. Johnson-Greene D. Dementia rating scale-2 (DRS-2): By P.J. Jurica, C.L. Leitten, and S. Mattis: psychological assessment resources, 2001. Arch Clin Neuropsychol 2004;19(1):145–7.
30. Garcia C, Leahy B, Corradi K, et al. Component structure of the repeatable battery for the assessment of neuropsychological status in dementia. Arch Clin Neuropsychol 2008;23(1):63–72.
31. Folstein MF, Folstein SE, McHugh PR. "Mini-mental state". A practical method for grading the cognitive state of patients for the clinician. J Psychiatr Res 1975; 12(3):189–98.
32. Kalish VB, Gillham JE, Unwin BK, et al. Delirium in older persons: evaluation and management. Am Fam Physician 2014;90(3):150–8.
33. Steis M, Fick D. Delirium superimposed on dementia accuracy of nurse documentation. J Gerontol Nurs 2012;38(1):32–42.
34. Richardson K, Fox C, Maidment I, et al. Anticholinergic drugs and risk of dementia: case-control study. BMJ 2018;361:K1315.
35. Yevchak A, Fick D, Kolanowski A, et al. Implementing nurse-facilitated person-centered care approaches for patients with delirium superimposed on dementia in the acute care setting. J Gerontol Nurs 2017;43(12):21–8.

36. Fick DM, Hodo DM, Lawrence F, et al. Recognizing delirium superimposed on dementia: assessing nurses' knowledge using case vignettes. J Gerontol Nurs 2007;33(2):40–7.
37. Hasemann WA, Tolson DW, Godwin J, et al. Nurses' recognition of hospitalized older patients with delirium and cognitive impairment using the delirium observation screening scale: a prospective comparison study. J Gerontol Nurs 2018; 44(12):35–43.

# Considerations for the Care of Transgender Individuals

Brittany Abeln, BSN, RN*, Rene Love, PhD, DNP, PMHNP-BC, FNAP

## KEYWORDS

- Transgender • Primary care • Treatment • Transgender care • Transinclusive care
- Transgender youth • Gender dysphoria

## KEY POINTS

- There are numerous health disparities faced by the transgender population. These gaps can be improved through the integration of transinclusive care in health care.
- An understanding of potential gender-affirming treatments and surgeries allows for an improvement of care in physical examination.
- An understanding of special considerations of the care of transgender youth is also important to improve outcomes.
- Increasing transinclusive care in the health care setting and reducing transgender-related discrimination in the health care setting aims to reduce the health disparities experienced by the transgender population.

The term transgender describes the experience of an individual whose gender identity does not match the sex they were assigned at birth.[1] Approximately 1 million individuals in the United States identify as transgender.[2] With this portion of the population identifying as transgender, it is important to contextualize and understand their experiences and health needs to ensure best patient outcomes. As transgender individuals are seen in all aspects of health care, it is critical that providers are prepared to care for this population.

## BACKGROUND/SIGNIFICANCE

As a population, transgender individuals are at an increased risk of experiencing health disparities. For instance, transgender individuals have disproportionate rates of HIV compared with the cisgender population (cisgender describes the experience of one's gender identity matching the sex one was assigned at birth).[3] The increased incidence of HIV in transgender individuals is because of a multitude of factors, but likely is a combination of poor access to services, engaging in sex work, and

Disclosure: There are no commercial or financial relationships to disclose.
University of Arizona, College of Nursing, 1305 N Martin Avenue, PO Box 210203, Tucson, AZ 85721-0203, USA
* Corresponding author.
*E-mail address:* babeln@email.arizona.edu

unprotected sex.[4] In addition, transgender adults have high rates of substance abuse and experience higher rates of depression than the cisgender population.[5,6] Transgender individuals report excessive alcohol use (21.5%) and cannabis use (24.4%).[5] They also report higher rates of depression—transwomen (24.3%), transmen (31.1%), and gender nonconforming individuals (38.2%) versus cisgender women (21.2%) and cisgender men (12.5%).[6] The increased rates of mental health inequalities can be attributed to the psychosocial issues often experienced by this population.[4] In combination with the aforementioned health inequalities, transgender individuals also experience transgender-related discrimination in the health care setting which ultimately affects their ability to receive quality care.[7] Transgender-related discrimination may keep this population from seeking care or lead to delays in seeking care.[7] The health inequalities experienced by the transgender population demonstrate the importance and need for change in the health care system to improve the quality of care.

A nationwide needs assessment of transgender individuals established the need for improvement in care in the primary care setting.[8] Of the transgender participants, 60% reported having a regular primary care provider.[8] Although this is still the majority, it is only a slight one. Only 43% of participants reported telling their primary care provider they were transgender.[8] This statistical is of special concern because the lack of disclosure to their primary care provider increases the risk for receiving substandard care. If the provider is unaware of the patient's identity, they will be unable to provide an adequate assessment or meet the psychosocial needs of the patient. However, some transgender individuals may choose to keep their transgender identity from their primary care provider based on concerns of safety or discrimination which ultimately further perpetuates health disparities. For those who chose to self-disclose, 20% of participants reported that they had to educate their providers on their own health care needs indicating gaps in provider knowledge.[8] The results from the needs assessment demonstrates the importance of understanding the experiences of transgender individuals to allow for the creation of an optimal primary care patient setting.

Other health inequalities experienced by this population include the lack of inclusivity in health care for transgender individuals, which contributes to feelings of alienation from their provider and to delays in care. If transgender individuals feel alienated from their provider, they may be less likely to seek care. To combat feelings of alienation, providers need to have an understanding of culturally competent transgender terminology and best practice recommendations. By using culturally competent terminology and providing evidence-based care, providers will ultimately improve health disparities in the transgender population.

## DISCUSSION
### Transgender Terminology

To provide transinclusive care, an understanding of transgender terminology and definitions is needed. **Table 1** provides basic definitions for culturally competent transgender terms.[1,8,9] The included terms function to provide basic knowledge and understanding of the experiences of transgender individuals. Understanding these terms will better prepare providers to care for this population.

**Table 1** provides culturally competent terminology that serves to promote understanding of the experience of transgender individuals. Primarily, it is the key to understanding the differences between sex and gender in relation to the transgender experience. Sex refers to how individuals are designated based on anatomic

**Table 1**
**Transgender terminology and definitions**

| Term | Definition |
|---|---|
| Sex | The anatomic and biological designation assigned to individuals when born |
| Gender | A person's outward expression of identity; the behaviors, expression, and roles associated with male or female identities |
| Transgender | An individual whose gender identity does not match the sex they were assigned at birth. A transgender man has a male gender identity but was assigned female at birth. A transgender woman has a female gender identity but was assigned male at birth |
| Gender dysphoria | The discomfort or stress caused by the experience of one's gender identity not matching the sex one was assigned at birth. Important to note that this may not be experienced by every transgender person. Transgender individuals may also experience it differently on a spectrum (that is more or less destructive or distressing). May be experienced at such a level to merit diagnosis via the Diagnostic Statistical Manual of Mental Disorders (DSM). However, transgender individuals are not inherently disordered |
| Nonbinary | A person who does not identify on the gender binary of male or female. Also known as gender queer, gender nonconforming, or gender fluid. Important to note that it is the individual who does or does not define themselves and as such it is from the individual that they should be identified |
| Transsexual | This is an umbrella term for transgender that is not often used, recognized, or accepted. However, some individuals may still choose to identify with this term |
| Cisgender | An individual whose gender identity matches the sex they were assigned at birth |
| Transinclusive | A term that encapsulates the inclusion of transgender individuals. In the health care setting, this means through the use of transinclusive forms, language, and documentation |
| Sexual orientation | As a term is separate from gender identity. Describes the sexual attraction of one individual to another |
| Transmasculine | Another identifying term for transmen who were assigned female at birth but identify as male |
| Transfeminine | Another identifying term for transwomen who were assigned male at birth but identify as female |
| Misgender | A term that describes the experience of identifying someone as the incorrect gender |

*Data from* Refs.[1,8,9]

differences at birth, whereas gender relates to one's outward expression.[1,8,9] It is when one's sex and gender identity do not match that they may identify as transgender.[1,8,9]

Gender dysphoria is also included in **Table 1**, but merits further discussion because it is a complex topic. It is important to understand what gender dysphoria means in the context of diagnosis in the Diagnostic and Statistical Manual of Mental Disorders (DSM-V). It is also important to understand that not all transgender individuals meet the diagnosis of gender dysphoria.

### Gender Dysphoria as a Diagnosis

As described in **Table 1**, gender dysphoria is the feeling of discomfort in the mismatch between one's gender identity and sex assigned at birth.[8] It is important for providers to understand the implications of gender dysphoria. Gender dysphoria is present in the DSM-V, but as with all transgender experiences it should not be pathologized.[8] It occurs when the symptoms of gender dysphoria become debilitating to the level of a mental disorder that merits formal diagnosis.[8]

A key feature of gender dysphoria as defined in the DSM, is a desire to be the opposite gender from the sex one was assigned at birth.[10] An additional key feature is the desire to have the primary and/or secondary sex characteristics of the opposite gender.[10] There are differences between the diagnosis of gender dysphoria in adults and in children, but similarly the feelings must last for at least 6 months.[10] It is important to also clarify that, according to the American Psychological Association, some transgender individuals may not have gender dysphoira.[10] Gender dysphoria is not in and of itself inherent to a transgender identity.[10]

It is also important to discuss the controversy attached to having gender dysphoria as a diagnosis in the DSM-V. Many transgender individuals find the inclusion of gender dysphoria in the DSM-V problematic because it potentially pathologizes their identity.[8] This feeling is reminiscent of when homosexuality was present in the DSM. This is because the diagnosis of gender dysphoria is tied into the individual's identity.[8] However, there are instances in which gender dysphoria becomes a debilitating mental disorder and merits treatment as such, which is why providers should be aware of the diagnostic criteria.

### Potential Gender-Affirming Treatments and Surgeries

It is important to clarify that not all transgender individuals will choose gender-affirming treatments and/or surgeries, which does not make them any more or less transgender.[11,12] In addition, this may be related to an inability to afford gender-affirming treatment and/or surgeries.[11] The timeframe (adolescence versus adulthood) in which transgender individuals seek gender-affirming treatment and/or surgeries will also affect what options may be available to them.[8] An overview of potential gender-affirming treatments and surgeries is discussed in **Tables 2** and **3**.[8,9] Even though only expert providers will likely oversee this treatment, an understanding of the array of

| Table 2 | |
| --- | --- |
| **Gender-affirming surgical interventions in transmen** | |
| **Surgical Intervention** | **Description** |
| Phalloplasty/ scrotoplasty | A surgical procedure that creates a penis via a multitude of surgical options—commonly with a skin flap. Occurs commonly after a hysterectomy and vaginectomy. Erectile implants can be used to allow for increase in sexual function. Colloquially referred to at times as "bottom surgery" <br> Risks: infection, wound contraction, dysuria |
| Mastectomy | Involves the removal of the breast tissue to construct a masculine chest. Colloquially referred to as "top surgery" Important that transmen are still properly assessed for breast cancer because they have higher incidence because of poor screening guidelines <br> Risks: infection, scarring, nipple graft complications |

*Data from* Deutsch MB. Guidelines for the Primary and Gender-Affirming Care of Transgender and Gender Nonbinary People. Center of Excellence for Transgender Health, Department of Family and Community Medicine, University of California San Francisco. 2016. Available at: www.transhealth.ucsf.edu/guidelines and World Professional Association for Transgender Health (WPATH). Standards of Care Version 7. Available at: wpath.org/publications/soc.

**Table 3**
**Gender-affirming surgical interventions in transwomen**

| Surgical Intervention | Description |
| --- | --- |
| Vaginoplasty | Involves the creation of a vagina through various techniques, most commonly penile inversion. Dilation must be performed by the patient to ensure the integrity of vagina<br>Risks: infection, fistulas, urinary tract infections |
| Mammoplasty | Entails the placement of breast implants<br>Risks: infection |
| Facial feminization surgery | Involves a myriad of potential facial surgical procedures. Up to the patient which procedures they would like to have performed<br>Risks: infection, scarring |

Data from Deutsch MB. Guidelines for the Primary and Gender-Affirming Care of Transgender and Gender Nonbinary People. Center of Excellence for Transgender Health, Department of Family and Community Medicine, University of California San Francisco. 2016. Available at: www.transhealth.ucsf.edu/guidelines and World Professional Association for Transgender Health (WPATH). Standards of Care Version 7. Available at: wpath.org/publications/soc.

options is important. In the health care setting, providers should be prepared to refer out to specialists for their transgender patients seeking gender-affirming treatments and/or surgeries.[8]

Surgical treatments come with various pros and cons and additionally may not be undertaken by transgender individuals.[8] To reiterate—the choice to have or not have a treatment/surgery does not make an individual more or less transgender.[8] Transmen may choose to have a phalloplasty/scrotoplasty and/or a mastectomy.[8] These surgical interventions are outlined in **Table 4**. Transwomen individuals may

**Table 4**
**Recommendations for transinclusive language**

| Recommendation | Example/Explanation |
| --- | --- |
| Be respectful | "Welcome! What is your name and appointment time?"<br>No need to assume gender of the patient by saying sir/ma'am. A welcoming statement that allows individual to tell staff their name and elaborate if different from their preferred name is appropriate |
| Ask pronoun or name preference if unsure | "What name and pronouns do you prefer?"<br>Important to clarify with patient as electronic health record or charting may not accurately reflect their identity or preferences |
| Only ask necessary information | It is important that an accurate surgical/health history is ascertained, but also important that for patient's privacy only questions relevant to the visit are asked |
| Apologize if mistake in pronoun or name is made | "I am sorry [correct name or pronoun]. That will not happen again"<br>If the wrong name or pronoun is used, correct the mistake and apologize, recognizing how painful misgendering can be |
| Use gender inclusive language | Instead of "his" or "hers" use "theirs"<br>Instead of "man" or "woman" use "person" |

Data from Deutsch MB. Guidelines for the Primary and Gender-Affirming Care of Transgender and Gender Nonbinary People. Center of Excellence for Transgender Health, Department of Family and Community Medicine, University of California San Francisco. 2016. Available at: www.transhealth.ucsf.edu/guidelines and World Professional Association for Transgender Health (WPATH). Standards of Care Version 7. Available at: wpath.org/publications/soc.

elect to have a vaginoplasty, mammoplasty, and/or facial feminization surgery.[8] The decision to undergo or not undergo all the aforementioned surgeries is strictly up to the individual.

In terms of medical/nonmedical interventions, there are various options for transgender individuals. The primary medical treatment that many people choose is hormone therapy to acquire gender-affirming secondary sex characteristics.[8] Nonmedical interventions might range from hair removal to voice modification/training to genital tucking or packing to chest binding.[8,9] Knowledge and understanding of various medical treatments and/or surgeries that transgender patients may choose ultimately may affect the physical examination, but before the patient undergoes a physical examination it is crucial a transinclusive environment is created.

### Creating a Transinclusive Environment

A transinclusive environment in the health care setting is critical to ensure that transgender individuals feel welcome while also decreasing transgender-related discrimination.[8,9] There are many details to consider when creating a transinclusive environment. It is important for the waiting area, bathrooms, and forms be considered. The language that both staff and provider use is crucial as well.

First, consider the waiting area because this is the individual's first interaction with the health care setting[8,9] Waiting areas can be made transinclusive through the use of posters, brochures, and staff training.[8,9] Posters in the waiting area can be used to demonstrate the office as a safe space for transgender individuals.[9] Brochures among all patient education materials can be included specifically focusing on transgender health.[9] Front desk staff should also be trained on the culturally competent transgender terminology as described in **Table 1**, as well as how to use that language to inclusively interact with transgender patients.[8,9] Inclusively interacting with transgender patients involves asking what pronouns they prefer to be called without making assumptions.[8,9]

Gender neutral bathrooms should be used to further create a transinclusive environement.[8] Rather than a sign indicating patients should use the bathroom of the gender in which they identify, gender neutral bathrooms are inclusive of nonbinary individuals who may not feel comfortable in a female- or male-identified bathroom.[8]

Transinclusive forms should also be used in the primary care setting.[8,9] Making forms transinclusive involves asking the patient to not only identify which sex they were assigned at birth (male or female), but also offers the selection of gender identity.[8,9] Sex assigned at birth should be indicated on the form with male or female options as well as gender identity (eg, male, female, transman, transwoman).[8,9] Furthermore, the addition of a nondiscrimination statement in health care forms supports a transinclusive environment.[8,9] A nondiscrimination statement demonstrates that the health care setting is inclusive of all identities. It also ensures individuals feel safe to receive care.

**Table 4** details best practices for transinclusive language to be used in the health care setting.[8,9] It is a great starting point for staff training on transinclusivity. It provides examples of language recommendations with accompanying explanations.

Demonstrating a transinclusive environment in the health care setting ensures the patient feels safe and welcomed. It also ensures that the patient feels more comfortable going into the physical examination. An understanding of considerations for transgender patients in the health care setting will ultimately lead to best patient outcomes and bridge the gap on health disparities.

### The Physical Examination

When conducting a physical examination with a transgender patient, it is crucial that a conversation occur with the patient beforehand.[8,9] The provider should ascertain the patient's comfort/discomfort and take the time to discuss the plan for the examination before beginning.[8,9] The medical and surgical history as needed to inform the examination should also be completed before beginning.[8,9] The provider should ask permission to touch the patient throughout the examination and explain every step.[8,9] Only relevant and necessary parts of the body to the assessment should be examined (ie, if the patient is complaining of knee pain, no need to examine chest).[8,9] The provider should also ensure privacy throughout the examination and that the patient is covered to their comfort level.[8,9] Throughout the provider's assessment they should be sensitive to both the needs and the responses of the patient.

### Special Considerations for the Care of Transgender Youth

The care and treatment of transgender youth is a growing field and as such it is important for providers to be aware of considerations for the care of this population.[8] Feelings of gender dysphoria most often present before puberty.[8] These feelings often intensify during adolescence and the development of secondary sex characteristics.[8] As the care and treatment of gender-affirming care in transgender youth is a complex process, referral to experts in clinical care is key.[8] Referral is needed when transgender youth wish to undergo gender-affirming treatments.[8] Consent for gender-affirming treatment must come from one or both parents, which can bring up additional challenges when consent is not present.[8] Often care involves using hormone blockers—gonadotropin-releasing hormone analogs—during the early stages of puberty to prevent the development of secondary sex characteristics followed by the use of gender-affirming hormone therapy.[8] Gender-affirming surgical treatment is more rare in youth and often takes place once the individual is older than 18 years of age.[8]

It is critical that mental health support and screening be offered for transgender youth as they are at an increased risk for mental health inequalities.[8] Transgender youth have higher rates of suicidal ideation compared with their cisgender peers.[13] An examination of within-group variation of transgender youth although a secondary data analysis with 120,617 participants examined suicide attempts.[14] The highest rates of suicide attempts were in female to male transgender adolescents (50.8%), followed by nonbinary adolescents (41.8%), male to female transgender adolescents (29.9%), questioning adolescents (27.9%), female adolescents (16.6%), and male adolescents (9.8%).[14] Owing to the higher rates of suicidality in transgender youth, it is critical that suicide ideation be screened in the health care setting.[8] Providers should ask if the transgender youth have any thoughts of hurting themselves.

Providers support is also important during this process. It is important for families to have an accepting response to contribute to optimal outcomes for the adolescent.[8] Additional support can be provided through a referral to a mental health provider. This is also important in terms of the social transition of the youth in that they begin to present as the gender in which they identify, change their preferred pronoun and their name.[8] Mental health experts can assist in offering counsel and support to the families.[8] In addition, they can aid in the discussion of timing and the process of social transition.[8]

### Mental Health for the Adult Transgender Population

As discussed previously, there is a higher incidence of mental health inequalities in transgender youth. In addition, this higher rate of mental health disparities is also

seen in transgender adults. Owing to the mental health inequalities experienced by transgender individuals, it is critical that mental health assessment considerations are included in the health care setting.[6,13,14] General screenings for anxiety, depression, and suicidal ideation should be provided to transgender patients and, if needed, a referral to a mental health provider when needed.[6,13,14]

Gender dysphoria should be assessed in transgender individuals by a mental health provider.[8,9] As previously outlined, gender dysphoria may not be present in all transgender individuals.[8,9] Referrals for medical intervention and gender-affirming treatment should also be made to experts in those fields to assist in improving mental health outcomes.[8,9] It is also important to assess coexisting mental health concerns, such as anxiety and depression and ensure those concerns are treated.[8,9]

Family therapy and support is also important and should be encouraged when family members are involved.[8] A secondary data analysis found that family rejection increased the rate of substance abuse and suicide attempts in transgender individuals.[15] If providers have access to family members they should assess support levels, because individuals with less support may be especially vulnerable.[8,15] Providers should also recognize their role of education and advocacy for the transgender population out in the community to assist in improving social support in the community.[8]

## SUMMARY

Transgender individuals are especially vulnerable because of the numerous health inequalities they face. It is critical that improvements be made in the health care setting to improve outcomes and to better prepare providers to care for this population. An understanding of culturally competent transgender terminology better prepares providers to care for this population and reduces transgender-related discrimination in the health care setting. In addition, when providers have a knowledge of gender-affirming surgeries and treatments available to transgender individuals, they are better prepared to provide care and refer to specialists. Improvements in the care of transgender individuals in the health care setting will ultimately bridge the gap on health disparities seen in this population.

## REFERENCES

1. Human Rights Campaign. "Transgender FAQ." Human rights campaign. Available at: www.hrc.org/resources/transgender-faq. Accessed October 2018.
2. Meerwijk EL, Sevelius JM. Transgender population size in the United States: a meta-regression of population-based probability samples. Am J Public Health 2017;107(2):e1–8.
3. Herbst JH, Jacobs ED, Finlayson TJ, et al. Estimating HIV prevalence and risk behaviors of transgender persons in the United States: a systematic review. AIDS Behav 2008;12:1–17.
4. McCann E, Brown M. Vulnerability and psychosocial risk factors regarding people who identify as transgender. A systematic review of the research evidence. Issues Ment Health Nurs 2018;39(1):3–15.
5. Gonzalez CA, Gallego JD, Bockting WO. Demographic characteristics, components of sexuality and gender, and minority stress and their associations to excessive alcohol, cannabis, and illicit (noncannabis) drug use among a large sample of transgender people in the United States. J Prim Prev 2017;38(4):419–45.
6. Downing JM, Przedworski JM. Health of transgender adults in the US, 2014–2016. Am J Prev Med 2018;55(3):336–44.

7. Bradford J, Reisner SL, Honnold JA, et al. Experiences of transgender-related discrimination and implications for health: results from the Virginia Transgender Health Initiative Study. Am J Public Health 2013;103(10):1820–9.

8. Center of Excellence for Transgender Health, Department of Family and Community Medicine, University of California San Francisco. In: Deutsch MB, editor. Guidelines for the primary and gender-affirming care of transgender and gender nonbinary people. 2nd edition; 2016. Available at: www.transhealth.ucsf.edu/guidelines.

9. World Professional Association for Transgender Health (WPATH). "Standards of Care Version 7." WPATH, Available at: wpath.org/publications/soc. Accessed October 2018,

10. American Psychiatric Association. Diagnostic and statistical manual of mental disorders. 7th edition. Arlington (VA): American Psychiatric Publishing; 2013.

11. Gay & Lesbian Medical Association (GLMA). Guidelines for care of lesbian, gay, bisexual and transgender patients. 2006. Available at: http://glma.org/_data/n_0001/resources/live/GLMA%20guidelines%202006%20FINAL.pdf. Accessed October 2018.

12. American Psychological Association. Report of the APA task force on gender identity and gender variance. American Psychological Association; 2009. Available at: www.apa.org/pi/lgbt/resources/policy/gender-identity-report.pdf.

13. Reisner SL, Vetters R, Leclerc M, et al. Mental health of transgender youth in care at an adolescent urban community health center: a matched retrospective cohort study. J Adolesc Health 2015;56(3):274–9.

14. Toomey RB, Syvertsen AK, Shramko M. Transgender adolescent suicide behavior. Pediatrics 2018;142(4):e20174218.

15. Klein A, Golub SA. Family rejection as a predictor of suicide attempts and substance misuse among transgender and gender nonconforming adults. LGBT Health 2016;3(3):193–9.

# Postpartum Depression
## Are You Listening?

Sophia D. Falana, BSN, RN*, Jane M. Carrington, PhD, RN

### KEYWORDS

- Postpartum depression • PPD • Treatment option for PPD
- Non–mental health providers PPD

### KEY POINTS

- Postpartum depression (PPD) affects 10% to 20% of women within the first year after birth and 25% beyond the first year.
- The assessment can be done using interview or patient assessment or administration of the Edinburgh Postnatal Depression Scale or Patient Health Questionnaire-2.
- Women experiencing PPD can have pharmacologic, nonpharmacologic, or combined treatment options.

## INTRODUCTION

Postpartum depression (PPD) or pregnancy mood disorder affects 10% to 20% of women within the first year after birth and 25% beyond the first year.[1] Often described as "baby blues," PPD is defined as a "major depressive episode" by experts and listed in the American Psychiatric Association's *Diagnostic and Statistical Manual of Mental Disorders, Fifth Edition (DSM-V)*.[2] Women who experience PPD generally have their first symptoms during pregnancy or within 4 weeks after delivery of their infant.[3] Despite advances in diagnosis and treatment of psychiatric mental health disorders, PPD remains underdiagnosed and misunderstood. Two key issues perpetuate misunderstandings of PPD: timeliness of diagnosis and diagnostic tools. Women do not always display signs of PPD while in care for delivery of the infant and may not discuss mood shifts with their primary care provider at discharge and first post-delivery appointment. The purpose of this article was to identify the most effective means for assessment, detection, and treatment of PPD in mothers who are considered at risk.

Disclosure Statement: The authors have nothing to disclose.
The University of Arizona, College of Nursing, 1305 North Martin Avenue, Room 437, Tucson, AZ 85721, USA
* Corresponding author.
*E-mail address:* sfalana@email.arizona.edu

## ASSESSMENT AND DETECTION

Assessing women for PPD is challenging and begins during prenatal care and extends beyond postpartum care periods. During prenatal care, the provider should assess the new mother for risk factors of PPD. Risk factors include the following: genetic predisposition to depression before pregnancy (family diagnosis), depression or anxiety at any point in the mother's life or pregnancy, socioeconomic status (eg, low socioeconomic status), marital discord or divorce, other mental health diagnoses including substance abuse, weak or nonexistent support system, unwanted or unexpected pregnancy, and low educational levels.[4] After determining family history and history of the new mother, the provider should be aware during the prenatal interview that new mothers who present with 5 or more symptoms, such as anxiety, depression, a significant decrease in participation in desirable activities, sleep disturbance (beyond the care of the infant), feelings of worthlessness, appetite changes, decreased concentration, recurrent suicidal thoughts or homicidal thoughts, racing thoughts, or psychosis, to name a few, may warrant the provider to refer the patient for a mental health consultation or to gather more information on his or her patient.[5]

Along with interviews and physical assessment, established tools also can be used to aide in the diagnosis of PPD. A thorough search of the literature revealed 9 articles that described 2 PPD assessment tools: the Edinburgh Postnatal Depression Scale (EPDS) and the Patient Health Questionnaire-2 (PHQ-2). These are considered to be the most useful in the detection of PPD because of their sensitivity and specify. Each is further discussed in **Table 1**.

### Patient Health Questionnaire-2

The PHQ-2 has been widely validated and accepted in both primary and pediatric health care settings. It consists of only the first 2 questions from the well-known PHQ-9 questionnaire, a 9-question Likert depression questionnaire that was developed based on the diagnostic criteria for depression. The PHQ-9 assesses events from the past 2 weeks, including suicidal thoughts and attempts.[11] Questions are scored from 0 (being none) to 3 (the worst ever felt). A score of more than 10 or a positive response to suicide should result in further treatment and evaluation by a psychiatric mental health provider.[11]

### Edinburgh Postnatal Depression Scale

The EPDS is used more often than any other screening tool because of the ability to detect not only depression but also anxiety in patients.[12] EPDS is a widely used validated 10-question screening tool for both clinical and research settings, published in 1987, to detect depression in postpartum women. Unlike the PHQ-9, the EPDS screening tool assesses the frequency of symptoms in the past 7 days[4,13,14]; however, trying to find the appropriate cutoff point and when to screen mothers for PPD has not been established. Knight and colleagues[15] recommend the cutoff point to be greater than 10, thus making it possible to detect depression symptoms earlier because it assesses both minor and major depression symptoms. Also, making sure to assess mothers at discharge from the hospital seems promising. According to a study of 1154 mothers completed by Teissedre and Chabrol,[16] mothers who were screened at 2 to 3 days postpartum had scores that were highly correlated (0.59) to screenings conducted at 6 weeks after delivery. This finding further reiterates the recommendation given by Wisner and colleagues[17] in 2002 to have mothers assessed for PPD using the EPDS at hospital discharge before going home.

**Table 1**
**Postpartum depression assessment tools**

| Background | Structure | Scoring and Cutoff | Sensitivity | Specificity |
|---|---|---|---|---|
| Edinburgh Postnatal Depression Scale (EPDS) | | | | |
| Developed by Cox et al,[6] in 1987 to help identify women who were suffering from mood disorder after giving birth | 10-item self-reported questionnaire; assesses depression and anxiety symptoms in mothers after delivery.[4] Any positive reply for question 10 needs immediate attention because the question asks about self-harming. | Scoring each question from 0 (no symptoms) to 3 (the worst ever felt) with total maximum score of 30. Cutoff score of >10. | 96%[7] | 82%[7] |
| Patient Health Questionnaire (PHQ) | | | | |
| Developed by Kroneke et al[8] in 2003 based on the *Diagnostic and Statistical Manual of Mental Disorders, Fourth Edition* to detect major depressive disorder in patients, not specifically for postnatal mothers. | 9-item self-reported questionnaire assesses the severity of depression; however, the first 2 questions of the PHQ-9 creates the PHQ-2, a shorter version of the questionnaire: "Have you been bothered by little interest or pleasure in doing things? Have you been bothered by feeling down, depressed, or hopeless?" If positive findings, the provider administering the questionnaire should administer the longer version with 9 questions to seek further information of the patient's symptoms.[8] | Scoring each question 0 (being none) to 3 (being the worse) on the Likert scale. Anything ranging >10 with a maximum of 80 points warrants a diagnosis of depression and needs further evaluation, treatment, and education for this mood disorder.[9,10] A patient who is positive for question 1 or 2, which speaks about suicidal ideations, will automatically need a mental health consult.[10] | 100%[11] | 79.3%[11] |

*Data from* Refs.[4,6–11]

Here we recommend the use of the EPDS for the detection of PPD in new mothers. This, along with a comprehensive assessment, should be completed during prenatal and postpartum care periods. The EPDS is a very simple tool that any clinician can administer to clients, whether a pediatrician or an obstetrician and gynecologist; thus, increasing the number of mothers being screened at a wellness visit.[4] Once a new mother is found to be at risk or is diagnosed with PPD, the effective treatment is required to support the health and well-being of the mother and infant.

## RECOMMENDATIONS FOR TREATMENT

After detecting PPD in mothers, whether assessing on discharge from the hospital or in the outpatient setting, it is important for providers to refer any patient deemed high risk (ie, score >10 using either instrument) to a mental health provider for further treatment. If the patient reports suicidal thoughts or attempts on her own life, it is the provider's responsibility to find transportation for that patient to the nearest emergency department for immediate treatment without delay, thus ensuring the mother is no longer left alone until she is deemed safe to herself and others by a provider. If the mother scored less than 10 on either assessment, then the mother is safe to be released home with PPD discharge instructions that includes signs and symptoms, as well as when to seek further assistance. Once PPD has been detected by clinicians, it is recommended that the mother is referred to a psychiatrist–mental health professional for treatment consisting of 2 goals: health and well-being of the mother and care and nurturing of the infant.

Two forms of treatment currently exist for PPD. First, the best available treatment when it comes to pharmacotherapy for PPD suggests that selective serotonin reuptake inhibitors (SSRIs), such as fluoxetine, rather than tricyclic medications are preferred for PPD treatment because of low or mild side effects; particularly sertraline, which has low or undetectable secretion amounts in the breast milk for mothers who want to breastfeed their infants.[18,19] Weighing the benefits with the risks when using sertraline or other similar SSRIs is important when initiating medications. A clinical trial of 22 mothers (sertraline, n = 14; placebo, n = 8) conducted by Wisner and colleagues[20] indicated that sertraline should be used for the first-line option for mothers in need of PPD treatment as well as breastfeeding mothers. It was noted that multiple laboratories confirmed the inability to detect the medication in infant blood serum levels and there were no reports of short-term adverse events in both mother and infant alike.[20] Although few side effects are identified, it is important to know that there is always a potential for side effects. Sertraline at a low dose of 25 mg/d, which is titrated up slowly, may particularly affect infants born prematurely or those with a low birth weight, which can be seen as irritability, difficulty sleeping or poor sleeping habits, and poor feeding.[20,21] Some side effects reported by mothers were headaches, nausea, and diarrhea with 93% compliance rate.[18] A mother should be educated to never stop medications without the assistance of a provider. Stopping medication always should be discussed with a health care provider so that medication can be changed or tapered. Stopping any medication abruptly will cause adverse reactions and side effects that are harmful to both the mother and the newborn. The mother should consider all risks versus benefits when it comes to medication treatment options for PPD. There are misconceptions about psychotropic medication and pregnancy that may affect a mother's compliance with medication recommendations.

Another form of treatment is nonpharmacological methods. Cognitive behavioral therapy (CBT) has shown promise for patients with PPD. Developed in the 1960s by Dr Aaron T. Beck, CBT is a psychosocial intervention.[22] The focus of CBT is challenging and ultimately addresses reframing of the patient's unhelpful thoughts and behavioral patterns.[22,23] Twelve weeks of CBT monotherapy has been deemed promising as a first-line therapy treatment option for PPD.

Some patients may benefit by both pharmaceutical and nonpharmaceutical treatment or a combined approach. In a recent study conducted by Milgrom and colleagues,[19] individuals who were compliant with the therapy session experienced a reduction in both anxiety and depression when given alone (monotherapy) as opposed to medication or combined treatment (medication and CBT). Both CBT monotherapy and psychotropic treatment with sertraline has allowed mothers to go into complete remission without the need for further treatment due to relapse.[19] On the other hand, compliance for treatment options reduced when both medication and therapy sessions were combined because of the time factor required for therapy sessions and medication management.[19] The increased burden of multiple appointments is deemed as a stressor for new mothers struggling with PPD, thus decreasing compliance rates as compared with those who did both treatment options separately. It is essential that the provider determine the best treatment option for the patient and work with the patient to increase compliance. Treatment should extend until the new mother experiences complete remission from PPD and is deemed safe.

## ROLE OF THE NURSE

To support the goal of Healthy People 2020 for increasing screening for depression in adults, nurses can help with intake screening and treatment or referral of the individual.[24] Nurses have the unique advantage of helping communities develop programs to help reduce the risk of PPD in low-income communities and by teaming up with organizations such as the Transdisciplinary Research Consortium for Gulf Resilience on Women's Health to ensure new mothers have the support needed for the first year, as well as the most effective treatment option if needed.

Another effective postnatal support using community health workers (CHWs) for 6 months postpartum was developed by Mundorf and colleagues.[25] The program decreased the risk for PPD for first-time mothers living in low-income communities compared with those without the support. The CHWs went to the mother's home daily at the beginning of the program and then decreased the visits as the mother became aware of how to balance her new life with a newborn. The CHWs taught the mother how to care for the newborn as well as herself, by acting as a support partner for the mother. Mothers at the end of the study reported that with the added support, they were less likely to develop PPD because they did not feel alone, and they knew their support person was coming to help relieve the stress or just help them balance their day.[25] The only difference in the study was seen when mothers and CHWs did not pair well. Assessing the mother and the CHW's relationship will be key for improvement in the mother's condition to advance this study beyond the Gulf coast.

## SUMMARY

Finding the best screening tool for the provider is key to help identify mothers with PPD. Teaching mothers how to not only care for their infants but also themselves is important as well. Mothers are always taught about feeding, changing, and bathing schedules. However, knowing the signs and symptoms of PPD and when and who to call for help is important on hospital discharge. Assessing a mother at hospital discharge will increase the likelihood of decreasing the 10% to 20% of mothers who go undetected until 6 months postpartum.[1]

## REFERENCES

1. Sriraman NK, Melvin K, Meltzer-Brody S. ABM clinical protocol #18: use of antidepressants in breastfeeding mothers. Breastfeed Med 2015;10:290–9.
2. American Psychiatric Association. Diagnostic and statistical manual of mental disorders. 5th edition. Arlington (VA): American Psychiatric Publishing; 2013.
3. Stewart DE, Vigod S. Postpartum depression. N Engl J Med 2016;375(22): 2177–86.

4. Mgonja S, Schoening A. Postpartum depression screening at well-child appointments: a quality improvement project. J Pediatr Health Care 2016;31(2):178–83.
5. Liberto TL. Screening for depression and help-seeking in postpartum women during well-baby pediatric visits: an integrated review. J Pediatr Health Care 2012; 26(2):109–17.
6. Cox JL, Holden JM, Sagovsky R. Detection of postnatal depression. Development of the 10-item Edinburgh Postnatal Depression Scale. Br J Psychiatry 1987;150:782–6.
7. Yawn BP, Pace W, Wollan PC, et al. Concordance of Edinburgh Postnatal Depression Scale (EPDS) and Patient Health Questionnaire (PHQ-9) to assess increased risk of depression among postpartum women. J Am Board Fam Med 2009;22(5): 483–91.
8. Kroenke K, Spitzer RL, Williams JB. The Patient Health Questionnaire-2: validity of a two-item depression screener. Med Care 2003;41(11):1284–92.
9. Flanagan T, Avalos LA. Perinatal obstetric office depression screening and treatment: implementation in a health care system. Obstet Gynecol 2016;127(5): 911–5.
10. Bennet IM, Coco A, Coyne JC, et al. Efficiency of a two-item pre-screen to reduce the burden of depression screening in pregnancy and postpartum: an IMPLICIT network study. J Am Board Fam Med 2008;21(4):317–25.
11. Chae SY, Chae MH, Tyndall A, et al. Can we effectively use the two-item PHQ-2 to screen for postpartum depression? Fam Med 2012;44(10):698–703. Available at: https://fammedarchives.blob.core.windows.net/imagesandpdfs/pdfs/FamilyMedicineVol44Issue10Chae698.pdf.
12. Guedeney N, Fermanian J, Guelfi JD, et al. The Edinburgh Postnatal Depression Scale (EPDS) and the detection of major depressive disorders in early postpartum: some concerns about false negatives. J Affect Disord 2000;61:107–12.
13. Wilkinson A, Anderson S, Wheeler SB. Screening for and treating postpartum depression and psychosis: a cost-effectiveness analysis. Matern Child Health J 2017;21(4):903–14.
14. Agency for Healthcare Research and Quality. Efficacy and safety of screening for postpartum depression. 2013. Available at: http://www.effectivehealthcare.ahrq.gov/ehc/products/379/1438/postpartum-screening-executive-130409.pdf.
15. Knights JE, Salvatore ML, Simpkins G, et al. In search of best practice for postpartum depression screening: is once enough? Eur J Obstet Gynecol Reprod Biol 2016;206:99–104.
16. Teissedre F, Chabrol H. Detecting women at risk for postnatal depression using the Edinburgh Postnatal Depression Scale at 2 to 3 days postpartum. Can J Psychiatry 2004;49:51–4.
17. Wisner KL, Parry BL, Piontek CM. Clinical practice. Postpartum depression. N Engl J Med 2002;347:194–9.
18. Hantsoo L, Ward-O'Brien D, Czarkowski KA, et al. A randomized, placebo-controlled, double-blinded trial of sertraline for postpartum depression. Psychopharmacology 2013;231(5):939–48.
19. Milgrom J, Gemmill AW, Ericksen J, et al. Treatment of postnatal depression with cognitive behavioural therapy, sertraline and combination therapy: a randomised controlled trial. Aust N Z J Psychiatry 2015;49:236–45.
20. Wisner KL, Perel JM, Peindl KS, et al. Prevention of postpartum depression: a pilot randomized clinical trial. Am J Psychiatry 2004;161(7):1290–2.
21. Cuomo A, Maina G, Neal SM, et al. Using sertraline in postpartum and breastfeeding: balancing risks and benefits. Expert Opin Drug Saf 2018;17(7):719–25.

22. Beck J. Cognitive behavior therapy: basics and beyond. 2 edition. New York: The Guilford Press; 2011.
23. Beck AT, Haigh EA. Advances in cognitive theory and therapy: the generic cognitive model. Annu Rev Clin Psychol 2014;10:1–24.
24. Office of Disease Prevention and Health Promotion. Healthy People 2020 maternal, infant, and child health objectives. 2016. Available at: https://www.healthypeople.gov/2020/data-search/Search-the-Data?f%5B%5D=field_topic_area%3A3492&ci=0&se=0&pop=#.
25. Mundorf C, Shankar A, Moran T, et al. Reducing the risk of postpartum depression in a low-income community through a community health worker intervention. Matern Child Health J 2018;22:520–8.

# Evidence-based Care of the Human Trafficking Patient

Christine B. Costa, DNP, PMHNP-BC[a],*,
Kathleen T. McCoy, DNSc, APRN, PMHNP-BC, PMHCNS-BC, FNP-BC[b],
Gayle J. Early, PhD, FNP-BC[a], Cathleen M. Deckers, EdD, RN[a]

## KEYWORDS

- Human trafficking • Biopsychosocial assessment • Trauma informed care
- Public health

## KEY POINTS

- The major underpinnings of human trafficking associated with occurrence in both adults and children need examination.
- The use of biopsychosocial assessment is imperative to identify at-risk patients and mental health needs resulting from trauma.
- Evidence-based pharmacologic and psychotherapeutic approaches are included in the treatment of trauma patients.
- The use of trauma informed care is an effective evidence-based approach to guide health care providers in-going education and treatment.

## INTRODUCTION

Human trafficking is now recognized as an emerging health care priority worldwide. Trafficking is a public health issue that requires the involvement of professionals in public health, social work, nursing, and direct clinical services as well as members of the government, task forces, legal, and law enforcement communities.[1] Primary care providers are well positioned to identify and assist trafficked individuals as well as those who may be at risk for exploitation. There is a growing need to understand the various forms of human trafficking that can be observed as well as the diagnostic considerations involved. Therefore, in order to better understand these elements, it is necessary to take a closer look at each of them individually.

The definition of human trafficking, also called trafficking in persons, includes the concept of movement of people, usually with the intent to smuggle them for one reason or another. Another key concept in human trafficking is that of modern-day

Disclosure Statement: The authors have no disclosures to report.
[a] California State University, Long Beach, School of Nursing, 1250 Bellflower Boulevard, Long Beach, CA 90840-0301, USA; [b] University of South Alabama, College of Nursing, 5721 USA Drive North HAHN 3044, Mobile, AL 36688-0002, USA
* Corresponding author.
*E-mail address:* Christine.costa@csulb.edu

slavery.[1] This slavery can take several different forms, including sexual servitude and forced labor.[2] Historically, human trafficking is difficult to accurately identify and predict, creating problems for law enforcement.

Human trafficking is the fastest-growing criminal industry in the world, with an estimated 27 million people enslaved worldwide; among these, between 14,500 and 17,500 people are trafficked into the United States every year.[3] The high prevalence of trafficking is related to its profitability for criminals. The United Nations has classified human trafficking as the third most profitable crime in the world, and the issue encapsulates several political, legal, and social elements within society.[4]

## DISCUSSION
### Forms of Human Trafficking

Sex trafficking and labor trafficking each has its own unique traumatic experiences. Both include deprivation of liberty and inhumane working conditions as well as unfair wage deductions and sexual assault.[5] A distinction between sex trafficking and labor trafficking exists because of the unilateral differences between clients, victims, and consequences. They are not exclusive, however, and other forms of human trafficking exist. One particularly common form of human trafficking is child labor. Child labor is prevalent across the globe.[4] **Table 1** reveals examples of the 2 major forms of human trafficking, sexual exploitation and forced labor.[5]

### Vulnerable Populations

Children are perhaps the most vulnerable population to human trafficking. They are frequently targeted, not only because of the ease of kidnapping but also because of

| Table 1 Major forms of human trafficking | |
| --- | --- |
| Sexual exploitation Involves adults and children | • Commercial sex industry<br>• Street-based, Internet-based, or brothel-based prostitution; pornography<br>• Coerced employment in sexualized jobs as hostesses, exotic dancers, strippers, escorts, massage parlor workers, or companions at truck stops<br>• Survival sex—trading sexual acts for shelter, food, drugs, or protection<br>• Mail order brides |
| Forced labor Bonded labor Child labor | • Person forced to work against his or her will under the threat of violence or other punishment; occurs in agriculture, landscaping, manufacturing, hospitality, janitorial and other service industries, restaurants, and domestic settings<br>• Labor demanded to repay a "debt" in which terms and conditions have not been defined or in which the value of the victim's services as reasonably assessed is not applied toward the liquidation of the debt, pay off an artificially inflated "debt" for transportation, training, housing, sustenance, or even "uniforms"<br>• May include additional roles, such as drug couriering, child soldiering, exploitative or slavery-like practices in the informal industrial sector; members of begging and peddling rings; and domestic servitude, which can be both physically and sexually exploitative |

*Data from* Davidson JO. Moving children? Child trafficking, child migration, and child rights. Critical Social Policy.2011; Aug;31(3):454-77.

their long-term value for those who purchase these victims. Children often are groomed for trafficking from a young age. Trafficking creates many concerns that are difficult for children to overcome. Children often are not given the protections they need to avoid becoming victimized and experiencing the harmful effects thereof. A growing trend in the trafficking of children is that it may not involve much movement. Children may be used in fringe situations, such as the arrangement of marriages and faking of travel documents, among others.[6] These situations can have unique and very harmful effects on the children. Health care providers must remember that they are mandated to report suspicions of child trafficking.

Women also are vulnerable to human trafficking and represent a major component of the sex element. Trafficked women often endure manipulation, abuse, shame, intimidation, and deportation. The stigma associated with sex work creates an additional layer of difficulty in admitting to abuse and engaging in treatment.[7] Another population that is vulnerable but less recognized is individuals who are marginalized in some way. This is exacerbated when the person who is marginalized happens to be female, a child, or both. The recruitment stage of human trafficking, wherein individuals receive deceptive offers in order to be exploited by traffickers, is when they are the most vulnerable. Those who are poor are among the most salient of vulnerable populations.[8] Human trafficking victims often are those who perceive they have no other options. Traffickers may act as intermediaries between vulnerable individuals and employers, because they are able to offer a product to these employers, in the form of the individual.[9] **Box 1** lists the most common populations vulnerable to trafficking.[8]

Among the risk factors for human trafficking, socioeconomic inequalities stand out as common factor for those who are trafficked. Individuals may see no alternative but to turn to human trafficking, as victims or as perpetrators of it themselves. This situation is one that frequently repeats in developing nations.[8] Signs that health care providers may observe in trafficked individuals are shown in **Box 2**.[9]

### Health Care Providers

Victims of human trafficking may be unable to find the care they need from health care providers.[10] This means that many victims simply deal with their own psychological issues. Health care providers should remember that every culture has a distinct perspective about mental health and beliefs about the benefits of seeking mental health services. Counseling, in general, is a predominantly western practice and in some cultures folk healing, healing rituals, and secret societies are the commonly

---

**Box 1**
**Vulnerable populations**

Impoverished

Pregnant

Homeless

Human immunodeficiency virus positive

Sex workers

Refugees

Transgender

Children

---

**Box 2**
**Signs of trafficked individuals**

Delayed presentation for medical care

Discrepancy between the stated history and the clinical presentation or observed pattern of injury

Scripted, memorized, or mechanically recited history

Stated age older than visual appearance

Subordinate, hypervigilant, or fearful demeanor

Inability to produce identification documents

Documents in the possession of an accompanying party

Reluctance or inability to speak on one's own behalf

Accompanying individual who answers questions for the patient or otherwise controls the pace and content of the encounter

Companion or accompanying individual who insists on providing translation

Companion who refuses to leave

Evidence of a lack of care for previously identified or obviously existing medical conditions

Tattoos or other marks or insignias that may indicate a claim of "ownership" by another

Evidence of any kind of physical violence, including torture

---

accepted forms of health care.[11] Health care providers should familiarize themselves with the beliefs, values, and practices of the various cultures of their patients, so they are able to provide culturally competent care.

### Culturally sensitive trauma-informed care

Culturally sensitive trauma-informed care is a framework for health care professionals to effectively provide trauma-informed assessment and intervention that acknowledge, respect, and integrate patients' and families' cultural values, beliefs, and practices.[12] One of the first steps in trauma-informed care is actively classifying these individuals as victims of human trafficking.[13] Once this has been done, it becomes easier to ensure that these individuals are able to receive the comprehensive help they need. **Box 3** outlines the steps of culturally sensitive trauma-informed care.

It is essential to evaluate the country of origin for the victim of human trafficking. Each country has its own unique human trafficking environment that must be considered in terms of appropriate interventions. It also is imperative to evaluate the impact of traumatic stress while highlighting survivors' strengths and supporting their resiliency. Many cultures do not differentiate psychological, emotional, and spiritual

---

**Box 3**
**Steps of culturally sensitive trauma-informed care**

- Recognizing variations in the subjective perception of trauma
- Restoring safety and re-establishing trust
- Attending to distress
- Working within and through the family

---

reactions from more physical reactions; rather, they focus on the impact of trauma on the body as a whole. Additionally, cultural factors influencing individuals' beliefs about threats and response to danger, which can play an important role in how individuals respond to violent crimes.[13]

### Comprehensive care

Practitioners need to screen and evaluate several areas to provide comprehensive treatment and hence need an understanding of trauma and trauma-related issues that victims experience in the present and over time. Areas for evaluation as part of comprehensive care are found in **Box 4**.

### Physical Considerations

Physical considerations include violence, particularly against women, as one of the most salient of physical issues when it comes to human trafficking.[14] Violence can take several forms, with rape the most prominent and potentially used as a way of controlling victims to remain silent. Among physical concerns are long-term injuries and deformities that may arise from the violence and squalid conditions experienced in human trafficking. **Box 5** lists possible physical injuries the trafficking victim may incur.

### Mental Health Considerations

Mental health disorders frequently arise as a result of human trafficking, and symptoms must be evaluated when considering the clinical presentation of human trafficking individuals across the lifespan.[1] Perhaps the most commonly occurring of these is posttraumatic stress disorder (PTSD).[15] Many suffer from PTSD in some form, which often intersects with physical issues, leading to a more complicated clinical presentation, such as brain damage.[16] PTSD may present as feelings of intense stigma, shame, anxiety, and hopelessness. Pathologic presentation may present with fear, panic attacks, sleep disturbance, dissociative disorders, and suicidal ideation. Over time, an individual with cumulative trauma presents with disrupted coping mechanisms.

### Social Considerations

For many, human trafficking is largely a social issue because it reflects the social values, or lack thereof, present within a society. One of the key considerations relates to prostitution. As many as 70% of women who are involved in prostitution are

---

**Box 4**
**Comprehensive care**

Primary care

Mental health care

Cancer screening

Violence and abuse screening

Substance abuse screening and treatment

Anticipatory guidance

Immunizations

Reproductive care

Dental care

> **Box 5**
> **Possible physical health injuries**
>
> Physical injuries—intentional and accidental burns; branding, tattoos, and other purposeful and permanent stigmata of ownership; blunt force trauma; firearm and knife wounds; strangulation injuries; fractures; dental and oral cavity injuries; traumatic brain injuries; neuropathies and other effects of torture; and scarring, especially from unattended prior injuries
>
> Exposure injuries—chronic back pain from repeated strain or overuse; vision and hearing impairment from lack of protective gear; skin, nervous system, and respiratory ailments from exposure to industrial or agricultural chemicals; effects of prolonged sun, heat, or cold exposure
>
> Reproductive injuries—rape or gang rape, genital trauma, repeated unwanted pregnancy, forced abortion, complications from repeated or poorly performed abortions, sexually transmitted infections (for example, chlamydia, gonorrhea, human papilloma virus, hepatitis B, hepatitis C, and HIV)

introduced to the commercial sex trade when they are adolescents, and human trafficking plays a major role in this.[17]

Several global considerations should be made in this regard. For instance, there are unique regional perspectives observed in different locations, for example, Asia, Europe, Eastern Europe, Latin America, Africa, and the United States.[18] Each of these regions has its own social implications for the long-term effects of trafficking. A practitioner must be able to understand how these regions work together in facilitating human trafficking. For this reason, a global approach is needed to understand human trafficking and trauma-informed care. Awareness of the multitude of possible conditions resulting from human trafficking helps ensure that the professionals involved are able to adapt and respond to a variety of situations.

### Assessment and Diagnosis of Trauma Patients

Several assessment and diagnostic considerations are indicated in the care of individuals traumatized by human trafficking. Diagnosis can be difficult due to the overwhelming number of problems commonly encountered. It also can be challenging to understand the short-term and long-term implications of many of these diagnostic considerations.[19]

### Screening domains

Screening domains include psychological reactions, specifically anxiety and depression, leading to feelings of hostility and self-harm, as well as physical sequelae, among other behavioral disturbances.[20] The diversity in screening that can be observed makes understanding these domains difficult. It may not be readily apparent which screening domain is most applicable. The victim of human trafficking may be affected by multiple overlapping ailments or issues.

An overgeneralization of these screening domains hampers the ability of individuals to receive appropriate treatment. Screening questions need to be posed for each of the primary domains and includes questions, such as "Is anyone hurting you?"[21] Questions such as these are important for understanding the innate issues affecting each victim of human trafficking and to better understand which screening domain is appropriate for an individual, thus streamlining the treatment. **Box 6** outlines the screening domains of human trafficking.

---

**Box 6**
**Human trafficking screening domains**

- Trauma-related symptoms
- Depressive or dissociative symptoms, sleep disturbances, and intrusive experiences
- Past and present mental disorders, including typically trauma-related disorders (eg, mood disorders)
- Severity or characteristics of a specific trauma type (eg, forms of interpersonal violence, adverse childhood events, and combat experiences)
- Substance abuse
- Social support and coping styles
- Availability of resources
- Risks for self-harm, suicide, and violence

---

### Screening instruments

A general, an open outlook is essential regarding screening instruments. The screening instruments used are immaterial in nature, but the key is long-term surveillance for specific signs of distress, especially in children, as well as psychological screening and basic medical care to prevent recurrence of self-harm.[22] It is important for practitioners to remain flexible and keep things simple when utilizing screening instruments.

A core component of screening is the degree of specificity used to ensure that victims are able to receive the help they need. Screening instruments should include ways to monitor and record the specific psychological issues facing an individual at any given time, allowing for an increased degree of insight into their unique needs. A goal of screening is to prevent victims' problems from becoming more damaging. In this regard, steps taken must focus on preventive care. Each component of screening must be considered carefully to ensure that there is a uniform level of understanding and treatment of human trafficking victims.[23]

Screening instruments should be able to help ameliorate many of the problems for trauma patients as well. These instruments must include medical staff training to better identify and understand the physical issues, training for psychologists, and other interdisciplinary professionals to increase the likelihood of detection and treatment.[24]

### Major components of a biopsychosocial examination

The biopsychosocial examination encapsulates psychological and social dimensions wherein an individual's thoughts and experiences become manifest. Through this, it becomes possible to formulate an in-depth understanding of their unique health needs.[25] The key component of the biopsychosocial examination is the interview itself. In the process, it becomes possible to formulate solutions to many of the problems (**Box 7**).

### Common Psychiatric Diagnoses and Clinical Presentations

The most common diagnoses for victims of trafficking are PTSD, panic disorder, and major depressive disorder. Each of these disorders presents several implications for prevention and treatment to decrease long-term functional impairments.[26] As discussed previously, PTSD often is correlated with human trafficking. In 1 study, approximately 55% of human trafficking victims met the diagnostic criteria for several mental

---

**Box 7**
**Major components of a trauma biopsychosocial examination**

Knowledge of physical health conditions

Engaging the client in the assessment process while maintain a safe environment

Assessing physical symptoms
- Evidence of acute or chronic trauma, especially to the face, torso, breasts, or genitals
- Bilateral or multiple injuries
- Evidence consistent with rape or sexual assault
- Pregnant woman with any injury, particularly to the abdomen or breasts; vaginal bleeding; or decreased fetal movement
- Occupational injuries not linked clearly to legitimate employment

Assessing a client's account of the presenting condition(s)
- How many hours per day (or week) do you work? What kind of time off do you have?
- Are you paid for the work you do? How much? Are you getting paid the amount agreed on?
- Can you come and go as you please during time off?
- Can you quit your job or situation if you want to?
- Have you been threatened with harm if you try to leave?
- Have you been physically or sexually harmed in any way by your employer or by an associate of your employer?
- Has anyone threatened or harmed your family?
- What are your working/living conditions like?
- Where do you live, sleep, and eat?
- Are there locks on the doors and windows where you work or sleep so you cannot get out?
- Do you have to ask permission to eat, sleep, or use the bathroom?
- Has your identification or documentation been taken away from you?
- Has anyone ever forced you to have sex when you did not want to?
- Have you ever exchanged sex for food, shelter, drugs, or money? Have you been required or forced to perform sex acts for work or to pay off a debt?
- Have you ever run away from home or from a program? What did you do in order to survive during that time?

Assessing psychological functioning
- Are you scared of or frightened by people in your everyday life or work setting?
- Do you feel that people are controlling you or forcing you to do things you don't want to do?

Assessing the impact of the physical condition on functioning

Assessing help-seeking and contact with, and treatment from, health professionals

Assessing the problem in the context of a client's system (support systems, legal, housing, and finances)

An increase in the frequency or severity of threats or assaults

Increasing or new threats of homicide or suicide by the trafficker if the patient discloses

The presence or availability of a firearm or other lethal weapon

New or increasingly violent behavior by the perpetrator

Assessing a client's resources and coping strategies
- Are you afraid to get help?
- Would you know how to seek help if you needed it?

Helping a client to articulate their aims for the intervention

Discussing the outcome of the assessment with a client

---

health disorders, in particular PTSD and depression, at 6 months after returning home.[27] PTSD can also develop as a result of complex trauma, generally arising not only from childhood sexual and/or physical abuse but also from trafficking, especially when sex is involved.[23] Human trafficking exposes the victim to a wide variety of traumatic experiences, and cumulatively these experiences often lead to PTSD and/or other psychiatric disorders.

### Posttraumatic stress disorder—International Classification of Diseases, Ninth Edition (Tenth Revision) 309.81 (F43.10)

To be diagnosed with PTSD, an adult must have all of the following for at least 1 month:

- At least 1 re-experiencing symptom—flashbacks, that is, reliving the trauma over and over, including physical symptoms like a racing heart or sweating, bad dreams, and frightening thoughts
- At least 1 avoidance symptom—staying away from places, events, or objects that are reminders of an experience; avoiding thoughts or feelings related to the traumatic event
- At least 2 arousal and reactivity symptoms—being easily startled, feeling tense or on edge, having difficulty sleeping, and/or angry outbursts
- At least 2 cognition and mood symptoms—trouble remembering key features of the traumatic event, negative thoughts about oneself or the world, distorted feelings like guilt or blame, and loss of interest in enjoyable activities
- Young children (less than 6 years of age)—these symptoms can include wetting the bed after having learned to use the toilet, forgetting how or being unable to talk, acting out the scary event during playtime, and being unusually clingy with a parent or other adult.
- Older children and teens: disruptive, disrespectful, or destructive behaviors; guilt for not preventing injury or deaths; and thoughts of revenge[28]

### Panic disorder—International Classification of Diseases, Ninth Edition (Tenth Revision) 300.01 (F41.0)

Panic frequently comes about by reliving a past experience, making it similar to PTSD.[23] There may be feelings of nausea, a detachment from reality, shaking, and dizziness.[29]

The prominent diagnostic criteria for panic disorder are recurrent unexpected panic attacks. Common features of panic attacks include an accelerated heart rate or pounding heart beats, chest pain, sweating, trembling, shortness of breath, a choking sensation, nausea, dizziness or light-headedness, numbness, chills or heat, a feeling of being detached from one's self, fear of losing control, and fear of dying. In addition to these attacks, there may be persistent worry or fear of having a panic attack and changing behaviors and routines to avoid attacks.[28]

### Obsessive-compulsive disorder—International Classification of Diseases, Ninth Edition (Tenth Revision) 300.3 (F42)

The disorder is characterized by intrusive and uncontrollable obsessions and compulsions that cause significant distress. Obsessions are thoughts, urges, or images that individuals experience as unwelcome and invasive. Obsessive-compulsive disorder (OCD) is a highly individualized disorder and people are more likely to experience obsessions when they are exposed to stressful situations.[30] In cases of childhood trauma, persons might respond with compulsions that they believe will prevent these events.

Both PTSD and OCD are characterized by recurrent and intrusive thoughts that are experienced as anxiety/fear inducing. As PTSD symptoms reduce, OCD symptoms increase, and, as OCD symptoms are treated, PTSD symptoms take over. OCD symptoms do not seem to replace the PTSD symptoms, but rather OCD symptoms are used to cope with, reduce, and avoid the trauma-related symptoms and memories.[30]

### Generalized anxiety disorder—International Classification of Diseases, Ninth Edition (Tenth Revision) 300.02 (F41.1)

Worry that is intrusive, excessive, debilitating, and persistent—lasting for more than 6 months. Fatigue, nausea, muscle tension, nervousness, sweating, irritability, and trembling are some of the physical symptoms. The level of concern is not in sync with reality and is greatly magnified with people realizing that their concerns are over-blown, but unable to decrease their anxiety.[28]

### Major depressive disorder—International Classification of Diseases, Ninth Edition (Tenth Revision) 296.3 (F33.0-F33.3)

Major depressive disorder is characterized by several emotional issues, primarily random feelings and occasional outbursts of intense sadness, as well as several fringe issues, including loss of interest in activities.[31,32] The result is a large degree of sadness and reliving of an experience; hence, trafficking can lead to the development or exacerbation of depression.

Signs and symptoms present most of the day, nearly every day, for at least 2 weeks, that indicate depression:

- Persistent sad, anxious, or empty mood
- Feelings of hopelessness or pessimism
- Irritability
- Feelings of guilt, worthlessness, or helplessness
- Loss of interest or pleasure in hobbies and activities
- Decreased energy or fatigue
- Moving or talking more slowly
- Feeling restless or having trouble sitting still
- Difficulty concentrating, remembering, or making decisions
- Difficulty sleeping, early-morning awakening, or oversleeping
- Appetite and/or weight changes
- Thoughts of death or suicide or suicide attempts
- Aches or pains, headaches, cramps, or digestive problems without a clear physical cause and/or that do not ease even with treatment

### Posttraumatic Stress Disorder Differential Diagnosis

The complex presentation of trauma patients can result in misdiagnosis. Therefore, it is important to carefully consider differential diagnosis of other mood and anxiety disorders due to overlapping symptoms with disorders, such as major depression, generalized anxiety disorder, and bipolar disorder. Borderline personality disorder has been diagnosed more frequently than PTSD because many of the symptoms overlap; these include a pattern of intense interpersonal relationships, impulsivity, rapid and unpredictable mood swings, power struggles in the treatment environ-ment, underlying anxiety and depressive symptoms, and transient, stress-related paranoid ideation or severe dissociative symptoms. The effect of this misdiagnosis on treatment can be particularly negative because clients with a borderline person-ality disorder diagnosis often are viewed as difficult to treat and unresponsive to treatment. A diagnosis of antisocial personality disorder may be made for men and women who have been traumatized in childhood, due to acting out behaviors, a lack of empathy and conscience, impulsivity, and self-centeredness, which all can be functions of trauma and survival skills rather than true antisocial characteristics. Finally, children and adolescents can be misdiagnosed as having attention-deficit/hyperactivity disorder due to impulsive behaviors and concentration problems.[31]

## Guiding Principles

Guiding principles for examining and treating a victim of human trafficking include

- Speaking to the patient alone
- Conducting a complete examination, with sexually transmitted disease screening, pregnancy test, and prophylaxis against sexually transmitted diseases, as indicated
- Evaluating and treating physical injuries
- Ensuring that follow-up care is established
- Taking steps to ensure patient safety by
  - Contacting law enforcement
  - Mandatory reporting of suspected abuse, neglect, or exploitation of minors or the disabled to the appropriate agency
- Providing community referrals for safe housing or shelters[29]

## Pharmacologic and Psychotherapeutic Considerations

### Pharmacologic interventions

There are several pharmacologic interventions possible to help ameliorate the symptoms of disorders commonly associated with human trafficking, including those of PTSD. They include treating sleep disturbances, such as nightmares and insomnia[33] (**Table 2**).

### Psychotherapeutic interventions

Psychological interventions need to address abuse and the potential for ongoing harm. It is essential to address stressors, such as housing, physical health, legal issues, and other relevant social stressors, prior to commencing trauma-focused psychological therapy. Techniques to regulate emotions and to cope with dissociation are an integral part of this therapy. Depending on an individual's need, there are psychotherapeutic interventions that can treat symptoms effectively, in particular depression, which is highly prevalent.[30] **Box 8** outlines a variety of psychotherapeutic interventions.

The mental health needs and treatment of individuals vary depending on their experiences and level of distress. Factors, such as cultural background, level of acculturation, and language, need to be considered because these factors may have an impact on treatment.[34,35] Providers who work with human trafficking victims should become aware of and competent in the use of cognitive therapeutic approaches to treat this population. Cognitive therapies have shown the best efficacy and are the preferred treatment to address the needs of human trafficking victims. The incorporation of other interventions, such as exposure, sleep hygiene, or rescripting therapy, should be made based on emerging research and in collaboration with the patients. Support groups must be carefully recommended based on patients and their issues related to fear and difficulty trusting others.[34]

### Legal considerations

A major source of victim advocacy for trafficked individuals remains health care professionals. Unfortunately, many health care professionals cannot identify trafficking victims presenting in everyday encounters. A majority lack an understanding of the

**Table 2**
**Pharmacologic interventions for posttraumatic stress disorder**

| Class or Action | Generic Names | Prescription Selection |
|---|---|---|
| Selective serotonin reuptake inhibitors | Paroxetine Fluoxetine Sertraline | First-line therapy for PTSD Fluoxetine and sertraline are given after a meal to avoid gastrointestinal disturbances and insomnia. Give paroxetine before bedtime because it usually causes sedation. |
| Serotonin-norepinephrine reuptake inhibitors | Venlafaxine | Similar effectiveness on PTSD symptoms Have shown to have little or no effect on nightmares and sleep difficulties and can increase these problems in some cases * Dose should be tapered very slowly to avoid discontinuation syndrome |
| Tricyclic antidepressants | Amitriptyline Desipramine | Better efficacy for insomnia and pain Shown efficacy with torture victims when few other therapies have been effective. Consider desipramine use for those with comorbid alcohol problems. |
| $\alpha_2$-Antagonist | Mirtazapine | Shown efficacy in PTSD Consider for patients with insomnia. |
| $\alpha_2$-Adrenergic blockers | Prazosin | Adjunctive treatment—$\alpha_1$-blockade Effective against insomnia and nightmares in PTSD |
| $\beta$-Blockers | Propranolol | Adjunctive treatment—$\beta$-blockage has effects on acute adrenergic PTSD symptoms. |
| $\alpha$-Adrenergic agonist | Clonidine | Shown to be effective against nightmares and hyperarousal |
| Antipsychotics | Risperidone Olanzapine Quetiapine | Atypical antipsychotics had an effect on intrusive symptoms but not against the avoidance or hyperarousal symptoms and also can be used as adjunct medication to selective serotonin reuptake inhibitors or serotonin-norepinephrine reuptake inhibitors. |
| Mood stabilizers (anticonvulsants) | Gabapentin Lamotrigine Topiramate | Has some effect on PTSD symptoms and can be tried when other medication is not tolerated |
| Mood stabilizers (anticonvulsants) | Valproic acid (histone deacetylase inhibitor) | Adjunctive agent with psychotherapy for PTSD |
| Benzodiazepines | Lorazepam Diazepam | Should be avoided but may be used in an acute setting for a short period of time * Avoid alprazolam because it has the highest chance of dependency. |

*Data from* Rauch SA, Cahill SP. Treatment and prevention of posttraumatic stress disorder. *Primary Psychiatry.* 2003; *10*(8), 60-65.

needs of victims and also lack appreciation of human trafficking as an endemic and local/regional reality. Guidelines are yet to be widely disseminated or integrated into health care professional curricula. Therefore, it is necessary to provide health care professionals with resources and additional training because legal insecurities are

---

**Box 8**
**Psychotherapeutic interventions**

Trauma focused cognitive-behavioral therapy—combines cognitive therapy with behavioral interventions, such as exposure therapy, thought stopping, or breathing techniques

Exposure therapy—aims to reduce anxiety and fear through confrontation of thoughts (imaginal exposure) or actual situations (in vivo exposure) related to the trauma

Eye movement desensitization and reprocessing—combines general clinical practice with brief imaginal exposure and cognitive restructuring (rapid eye movement is induced during the imaginal exposure and cognitive restructuring phases)

Stress inoculation training—combines psychoeducation with anxiety management techniques, such as relaxation training, breathing retraining, and thought stopping

Narrative exposure therapy—short-term evidence-based treatment of PTSD that was developed specifically for victims of multiple trauma; individuals are taken through their entire autobiography. Both traumatic and positive events are identified and understood within the wider sociopolitical context in which they occurred.

*Data from* Rauch SA, Cahill SP. Treatment and prevention of posttraumatic stress disorder. Primary Psychiatry. 2003; 10(8), 60-65 and Salami T, Gordon M, Coverdale J, et al. What therapies are favored in the treatment of the psychological sequelae of trauma in human trafficking victims?. J Psychiatr Pract. 2018; 24(2): 87-96.

---

**Box 9**
**National resources for health care providers**

**National Human Trafficking Hotline**: (888) 373-7888

https://humantraffickinghotline.org/

24/7—the hotline fields tips about potential trafficking situations, provides urgent and nonurgent referrals for services, and offers technical assistance and comprehensive antitrafficking resources.

**BeFree Textline**—text HELP to 233733 (BEFREE) to get help for victims or survivors of human trafficking or to connect with local resources

**Polaris Project**: national human trafficking resource center www.polarisproject.org/resources/tools-for-service-providers-and-law-enforcement

501C3 nonprofit supporting the national human trafficking hotline and providing resources for service providers and law enforcement (including health professional-specific training).

**Trafficking in Persons and Worker Exploitation Task Force** www.justice.gov/actioncenter/crime.html#trafficking

Hotline: (888) 428-7581, funded by the US Department of Justice; direct call to federal law enforcement from 9:00 AM to 5:00 PM EST on weekdays.

**National Center for Missing and Exploited Children**

www.missingkids.com/home

Hotline: (800) 843-5678, provides services, resources, training, and technical assistance to assist child victims of abduction and sexual exploitation, their families, and serving professionals.

**CyberTipline**

www.missingkids.com/CyberTipline

To offer leads and tips regarding suspected crimes of sexual exploitation committed against children.

another area that may be exploited by the human traffickers in order to manipulate the victims. This is especially true for illegal immigrants or when victims were originally lured out of a country and the trafficker took away documents. In these cases, the victims are persuaded that without documents they will not have any rights and may end up in prison or deported for violating immigration rules. At the same time, they persuade the victims that their sufferings will end after they work for the trafficker for a certain period of time. Victims of trafficking used for sexual exploitation are generally informed that if they try to escape they will be charged with breaking labor and prostitution laws and thus will be put in jail for many years with no possibility of escape. See **Box 9** for resources available for health care providers and trafficking victims in the United States.[36]

## SUMMARY

Health care providers need to be alert to possible signs of human trafficking, particularly among individuals of vulnerable populations, in order to identify, report, and treat victims. Awareness of culture is needed to understand how individuals seek assistance, define their problems, attribute psychological difficulties, experience their unique trauma, and perceive future recovery options. Culture also can directly influence individuals' outlook on their pain, expectations of treatment, and beliefs regarding the best course of treatment. In certain countries, it may be challenging to find a health care provider who has experience treating those who have been victimized by human trafficking. Therefore, it is important to ensure ongoing education on human trafficking.[37] Training is needed to increase awareness, encourage helpful responses, and inform primary care providers about available support options to ensure the mental health needs of trafficked individuals they may encounter.

## REFERENCES

1. Parreñas RS, Hwang MC, Lee HR. What is human trafficking? A review essay. Signs: Journal of Women in Culture and Society 2012;37(4):1015–29.
2. Brysk A, Choi-Fitzpatrick A, editors. From human trafficking to human rights: reframing contemporary slavery. Philadelphia: University of Pennsylvania Press; 2012.
3. Lee M. 1 Introduction: understanding human trafficking. In Human trafficking 2013 Jan 11 (pp. 13-37). Available at: https://www.ovcttac.gov/taskforceguide/eguide/1-understanding-human-trafficking/. Accessed September 1, 2018.
4. Winterdyk J, Reichel P. Introduction to special issue: human trafficking: issues and perspectives. Available at: https://doi.org/10.1177/1477370809347894. Accessed September 1, 2018.
5. Weitzer R. New directions in research on human trafficking. The ANNALS of the American Academy of Political and Social Science 2014;653(1):246–7.
6. O'Connell Davidson J. Moving children: child trafficking, child migration, and child rights. Critical social policy 2011;31(3):454–77.
7. Wheaton EM, Schauer EJ, Galli TV. Economics of human trafficking. Int Migr 2010;48(4):114–41.
8. Barner JR, Okech D, Camp MA. Socio-economic inequality, human trafficking, and the global slave trade. Societies 2014;4(2):148–60.
9. Abas M, Ostrovschi NV, Prince M, et al. Risk factors for mental disorders in women survivors of human trafficking: a historical cohort study. BMC Psychiatry 2013;13(1):204.

10. Barth J, Munder T, Gerger H, et al. Comparative efficacy of seven psychothera-peutic interventions for patients with depression: a network meta-analysis. Focus 2016;14(2):229–43.

11. Ottisova L, Hemmings S, Howard L, et al. Prevalence and risk of violence and the mental, physical, and sexual health problems associated with human trafficking: an updated systematic review. Epidemiol Psychiatr Sci 2016;25(4):317–41.

12. Dovydaitis T. Human trafficking: the role of the health care provider. J Midwifery Womens Health 2010;55(5):462–7.

13. Sue S, Zane N, Nagayama Hall GC, et al. The case for cultural competency in psychotherapeutic interventions. Annu Rev Psychol 2009;60:525–48.

14. Oram S, Stöckl H, Busza J, et al. Prevalence and risk of violence and the phys-ical, mental, and sexual health problems associated with human trafficking: sys-tematic review. PLoS Med 2012;9(5):e1001224.

15. Hodge DR. Assisting victims of human trafficking: strategies to facilitate identifi-cation, exit from trafficking, and the restoration of wellness. Soc Work 2014;59(2): 111–8. Available at: https://www.ncbi.nlm.nih.gov/pubmed/24855860.

16. Yakushko O. Human trafficking: a review for mental health professionals. Int J Adv Couns 2009;31(3):158–67.

17. Crane PA, Moreno M. Human trafficking: what is the role of the health care pro-vider? J Appl Res Child 2011;2(1):7. Available at: https://digitalcommons. library.tmc.edu/cgi/viewcontent.cgi?article=1033&context=childrenatrisk.

18. Shelley L. Human trafficking: a global perspective. Cambridge (United Kingdom): Cambridge University Press; 2010. Available at: http://demografi.bps.go.id/ phpfiletree/bahan/kumpulan_tugas_mobilitas_pak_chotib/Kelompok_7/Human_ Trafficking_a_global_perspektif_(Shelley).pdf.

19. Baldwin SB, Eisenman DP, Sayles JN, et al. Identification of human trafficking vic-tims in health care settings. Health Hum Rights 2011;13(1):e36–49. Available at: http://publichealth.lacounty.gov/ha/present/Staff_researchpapers/Susie_Baldwin_ Articles/BaldwinHHR2011.pdf.

20. Baldwin SB, Eisenman DP, Sayles JN, et al. Identification of human trafficking vic-tims in health care settings. Health Hum Rights 2011;13(1):e44.

21. Kiss L, Yun K, Pocock N, et al. Exploitation, violence, and suicide risk among child and adolescent survivors of human trafficking in the Greater Mekong Sub-region. JAMA Pediatr 2015;169(9):e152278.

22. Buller A, Vaca V, Stoklosa H, et al. Labor exploitation, trafficking and migran-thealth: Multi-country findings on the health risks and consequences of migrantand trafficked workers. Geneva (Switzerland): International Organization for Migration; 2015. Available at: https://publications.iom.int/books/labour-exploitation-trafficking-and-migrant-health-multicountry-findings-health-risks-and. Accessed October 27, 2017.

23. Author. Adult human trafficking screening toolkit and guide. Office on trafficking in persons. ACF Home, US Department of Health & Human Services. Geneva, Switzerland: International Organization for Migration; 2018. Webpage retrieved Sept. 2018 Available at: https://www.acf.hhs.gov/otip/resource/ nhhtacadultscreening.

24. Alonso Y. The biopsychosocial model in medical research: the evolution of the health concept over the last two decades. Patient Educ Couns 2004;53(2): 239–44.

25. Oram S, Abas M, Bick D, et al. Human trafficking and health: a survey of male and female survivors in England. Am J Public Health 2016;106(6):1073–8.

26. Oram S, Khondoker M, Abas M, et al. Characteristics of trafficked adults and children with severe mental illness: a historical cohort study. Lancet Psychiatry 2015; 2(12):1084–91.

27. Cloitre M, Courtois CA, Charuvastra A, et al. Treatment of complex PTSD: Results of the ISTSS expert clinician survey on best practices. J Trauma Stress 2011; 24(6):615–27.

28. American Psychiatric Association. Diagnostic and statistical manual of mental disorders. 5th edition. Washington, DC: American Psychiatric Association; 2013.

29. Dykshoorn KL. Trauma-related obsessive-compulsive disorder: a review. Health Psychol Behav Med 2014;2(1):517–28.

30. Beaulieu Robjant K, Roberts J, Katona C. Treating posttraumatic stress disorder in female victims of trafficking using narrative exposure therapy: a retrospective audit. Front Psychiatry 2017;8:63.

31. Belmaker RH, Agam G. Major depressive disorder. N Engl J Med 2008;358(1): 55–68.

32. Lipinska G, Baldwin DS, Thomas KG. Pharmacology for sleep disturbance in PTSD. Hum Psychopharmacol 2016;31(2):156–63.

33. Koirala R, Søegaard EG, Thapa S. Updates on pharmacological treatment of post-traumatic stress disorder. J Nepal Med Assoc 2017;56(206). https://doi. org/10.31729/jnma.3108.

34. Okech D, Hansen N, Howard W, et al. Social support, dysfunctional coping, and community reintegration as predictors of PTSD among human trafficking survivors. Behav Med 2018;44(3):209–18.

35. Lutz RM. Human trafficking education for nurse practitioners: integration into standard curriculum. Nurse Educ Today 2018;61:66–9. Available at: https:// www-ncbi-nlm-nih-gov.libproxy.usouthal.edu/pubmed/29175690.

36. Zimmerman C, Hossain M, Watts C. Human trafficking and health: a conceptual model to inform policy, intervention and research. Soc Sci Med 2011;73(2): 327–35.

37. Grace AM, Ahn R, Macias Konstantopoulos W. Integrating curricula on human trafficking into medical education and residency training. JAMA Pediatr 2014; 168(9):793–4. Cited Sept. 2018.

# Developmental Issues and Mental Health

Elizabeth Bonham, PhD, RN, PMHCNS-BC

## KEYWORDS

- Human development theories • Depression • Nursing • Mental disorders

## KEY POINTS

- How humans develop provides the foundation for our journey across the lifespan.
- Selected mental disorders include depression, anxiety, bipolar disorder, schizophrenia.
- Normal development helps the practitioner identify abnormal development.

How we develop as humans provides the foundation for our journey across the life-span. The trajectory of human development follows a course of milestones, benchmarks, and pathways. Considering the process of conception and subsequent in utero growth, we can observe fetal development to the extent we can assess infant weight and physical development. Technology, such as ultrasound sonography, once used for the most critical of maternal—infant problems, is a common and useful tool in discerning prenatal growth and development. We know through the work of pediatrician pioneers, such as T. Berry Brazelton[1] and Frances Ilg and colleagues[2] that infants have a developmental trajectory and generalizable behaviors. We know through the works of developmental psychology pioneers such as Piaget, Vygotsky, and Bronfenbrenner that there are cognitive, social, and ecological routes of progress for infants and children. Pioneers in policy, such as Marian Wright Edelman[3] advocated for compassionate and moral ways for families and communities to raise children so that healthy children became healthy adults. As biological and genomic research has brought us closer to understanding the brain, the etiology of mental illness is progressing from the psychodynamic origins postulated by Freud[4] to organic pathways and epigenetic derivations. The purpose of this paper is to discuss selected developmental theories and selected mental disorders in their relation to mental health.

## DEVELOPMENTAL THEORIES

Theories are created by scholars to guide research, administration, and practice. Human development theories have been postulated over time to explain and predict

Disclosure: The author has no relationships or conflicts with commercial companies to disclose.
College of Nursing and Health Professions, University of Southern Indiana, 8600 University Boulevard, Evansville, IN 47712-3534, USA
E-mail address: bethbonham@coopsone.com

human behavior. How humans develop, especially infants, was a source of inquiry for scholars such as Jean Piaget, a Swiss psychologist. How humans learn was a source of query for Lev Zygotsky, a Russian psychologist. Other developmental theorists such as Bowlby, Erickson, Skinner, and Kohlberg explored specific facets of human development. Furthermore, some scholars focused on specific developmental ages, such as White[5] who investigated the first 3 years of life. For this paper, 4 theories that provide theoretic foundations for human development that weave with mental health will be explored.

### Piaget and Cognitive Development

Piaget recognized that children develop at different rates but in an invariant sequence or, in the same order.[6] In addition, Piaget thought that although there was some biological influence involved, the development occurred not from a genetic specificity but from ways of thinking. As settings change, children—and adults!—try to make sense of the setting. Doing so requires assimilation, or taking in, accommodation, and organization. Using these processes, the child constructs her reality of the world and how to deal with it. This construction is done in relation to self, a link that triggers the notion of causality, or what is observed in the external world. Conversely, because the young self is without experience, she discovers external parts of the world before she understands self.[7] According to Piaget's first period of development, Sensori-Motor Intelligence (birth to 2 years), babies use organization to explore the external world through physical actions like grasping and hitting. This developmental period contains 6 stages: reflexes; primary, secondary and tertiary circular reactions; coordination of secondary schemes; and the beginnings of thought.[6] In this first period, children begin to sense what Piaget named object permanence, a process of finding a hidden object. However, although the child found the object in one place, she could not find it if it was hidden and moved to another place, a process Piaget called displacement. In the second period of Preoperational Thought (2–7 years) and the third period of Concrete Operations (7–11 years), children begin to use symbols and internal images in order to think. The thinking is disorganized and irrational demonstrated by the notion that dreams are external events (an explanation of nightmares) as well as egocentric, unclassified, and animistic (every object is living). As they get closer to 11, children begin to think more systematically by referring concretely to items and events. Piaget's fourth period of development of Formal Operations (11 to adulthood) realizes capacity for increasing abstract thinking and equilibrium where operations are perceived as interrelated and applicable. In summary, Piaget's theory emphasizes cognitive development occurs by making discoveries.

### Vygotsky and Social – Historical Learning

As a Marxist, Vygotsky believed that the context of social and historical environment took precedence when explaining human development.[6] Marxism espoused that humans developed and used tools for production that contributed to the common whole which Vygotsky promoted as a revolution in changes of psychology.[8] Vygotsky's theory regarding human development is one of constructivism; that is, the human uses environment and experience to interpret and construct his reality. Learning occurs contextually and actively rather than passively—the human is an active participant in his learning. In addition, Vygotsky's theory proposed a dialectical approach in that the more knowledgeable other has information or skill to teach to the human who is unaware or has not learned yet. The social interaction between the 2 creates a zone of proximal development (ZPD) which is where Vygotsky hypothesized learning occurred.[9] The ZPD is the distance between a student's ability to perform a task under another's guidance or collaboration and the student's ability to solve the problem independently. In this interaction, the guide is looking for the student's enthusiasm and perhaps articulation of his own learning. Application of Vygotsky's theory in education settings promotes active learning in contexts where students play an active role in learning. The roles of each may shift as one is learning and one is facilitating the learning therefore creating a reciprocal interface. To summarize, Vygotsky believed that social learning precedes development differing from Piaget's theory in which he proposed development necessarily precedes learning.

### Bronfenbrenner and Ecological Development

Urie Bronfenbrenner's theory of ecological human development presented a totally new way to explain human behavior. Rather than examining humans in a laboratory context, Bronfenbrenner postulated that the human develops in relation to her experiences with the environment.[10] The ecological environment is conceptualized as a nested structure named as mesosystem, exosystem, and macrosystem with the complex interactions within the settings being the microsystem. The linkages that the human has within the settings affects development. This interaction extends to the notion that development occurs or is affected by events within those settings where the developing human was not even present.[10] The ecology of human development theory is comprised of multiple definitions, propositions, and hypotheses. For example, Definition 1: The ecology of human development involves the scientific study of the progressive, mutual accommodation between an active, growing human being and the changing properties of the immediate settings in which the developing person lives… (p. 21). In addition, Proposition C states: If one member of a dyad undergoes developmental change, the other is also likely to do so. And finally, an example of Bronfenbrenner's hypotheses is Hypothesis 14: Human development is facilitated through interaction with persons who occupy a variety of roles and through participation in an ever-broadening role repertoire (p. 104). In summary, an ecological approach to human development requires systematic and extensive work to explore the relationship of the human and his environment from a developmental lens.

## BIOPSYCHOSOCIAL

The biopsychosocial model of development is relatively new and has been embraced by scholars and practitioners in social sciences such as nursing, social work and psychology because the model offers an exceptional holistic approach to human development. Traditionally, as humans presented with various symptoms of mental disorders, the symptoms were grouped into a disease and treated as a disease. This methodology could not consider other parameters of the human's life—for example, environment, social context, genetics, and more—which could very well be a major contributor to the symptoms. Eventually, psychiatry practitioners examined the human from a psychosomatic slant. Engel proposed that a new medical model would consider the cultural, social, and psychological in addition to the biomedicine presentation.[11] Although a scientific and rational approach assists human care, it became obvious that the human was more than a scientific, rational being. Indeed the biopsychosocial model is a way of understanding the complexities between physical and mental health care that can engage the practitioner and patient in a humane, unbiased, trusting, and participatory relationship.[12] The 4 selected theories for this paper and key features are summarized in **Table 1**.

**Table 1**
**Summary of key characteristics of selected developmental theories**

| Theory and Author | Key Characteristics |
|---|---|
| Cognitive Developmental Theory<br>Jean Piaget (1896–1980) | Sensori-motor intelligence<br>Preoperational thought<br>Concrete operations<br>Formal operations |
| Social Development Theory<br>Lev Vygotsky (1896–1934) | Social interaction<br>More knowledgeable other<br>Zone of proximal development |
| Ecology of Human Development<br>Urie Bronfenbrenner (1917–2005) | Person—roles<br>Structure—setting<br>Processes—mesosystem, exosystem, macrosystem |
| Biopsychosocial<br>George L. Engel (1913–1999) | Biological dimension<br>Social dimension<br>Psychological dimension<br>Behavioral dimension |

## MENTAL ILLNESS

In this section, 4 mental disorders are discussed. Although there are certainly many more disorders than those selected, these 4—depression, anxiety, bipolar disorder, and schizophrenia—were chosen because of their ubiquitous nature (ie, depression) or their devastating outcomes (ie, schizophrenia).

### Depression

Depression is the most common mental disorder in the United States and presents globally as one of the disorders that decrease years of life and increase years lived with disability.[13–15] Depression occurs across the lifespan and can arise from various situations (ie, post partum depression). More women than men are affected; more citizens aged 18 to 25 years (10.9%) are affected; and 4.3% of the American population has had at least 1 major depressive episode with severe impairment. These numbers translate into billions of lost dollars in income, lost days of employment, and contribute to the most undesired outcome of suicide. Common symptoms of depression in youth, adolescents, and adults can be seen in **Table 2**.

### Anxiety

Anxiety is the least diagnosed mental disorder but is one of the most debilitating. Anxiety occurs across the lifespan and interferes with school, job performance, and relationships. Anxiety disorders encompass a wide variety of presentations to include generalized anxiety disorder, panic disorder, and social anxiety. Another category of anxiety is phobia in which a person has an extreme fear about a specific thing or situation, that is, dogs with the fear causing significant distress and interference with daily life. Social anxiety is paralyzing and is manifest by fears of meeting or talking to people, avoidance of social situations, and few friends outside the family; the most debilitating social anxiety disorder may be agoraphobia. More women that men are affected; 31% of both adolescent and adult populations in the United States have had an anxiety disorder in the past year.[16] Common symptoms of anxiety can be seen in **Table 2**.

| Table 2<br>Selected mental disorders and symptoms | |
|---|---|
| **Mental Disorder** | **Common Symptoms** |
| Depression | • Feeling or appearing depressed, sad, tearful, or irritable<br>• Not enjoying things as much as they used to<br>• Spending less time with friends or in after school activities<br>• Changes in appetite and/or weight<br>• Sleeping more or less than usual<br>• Feeling tired or having less energy<br>• Feeling like everything is their fault or they are not good at anything<br>• Having more trouble concentrating<br>• Caring less about school or work or not doing as well in school or work<br>• Having thoughts of suicide or wanting to die |
| Anxiety | • Restless, keyed up<br>• Fatigue<br>• Difficulty concentrating<br>• Impending sense of doom<br>• Irritability<br>• Muscle tension<br>• Sleep disturbance<br>• Persistent, intrusive thoughts<br>• Repetitive behaviors<br>• Unable to control worrying |
| Bipolar disorder | *Manic* symptoms may include:<br>• Unrealistic highs in self-esteem—for example, a child or adolescent who feels all-powerful or like a superhero with special powers<br>• Great increase in energy<br>• Decreased need for sleep such as being able to go with little or no sleep for days without feeling tired<br>• Increase in talking—when the child or adolescent talks too much, too fast, changes topics too quickly, and cannot be interrupted<br>• Distractibility—the child's attention moves constantly from one thing to the next<br>• Thinking more quickly, for example, thoughts are on "fast forward"<br>• Repeated high risk-taking behavior, such as abusing alcohol and drugs, reckless driving, or sexual promiscuity<br>*Depressive* symptoms episode may include:<br>• Decreased enjoyment in favorite activities<br>• Low energy level or fatigue<br>• Major changes in sleeping patterns, such as oversleeping or difficulty falling asleep<br>• Poor concentration<br>• Complaints of boredom<br>• Major change in eating habits such as decreased appetite, failure to gain weight or overeating<br>• Frequent complaints of physical illnesses such as headaches or stomach aches<br>• Thoughts of death or suicide |
| Schizophrenia | • Seeing things and hearing voices which are not real (hallucinations)<br>• Odd and eccentric behavior and/or speech<br>• Unusual or bizarre thoughts and ideas<br>• Confusing television and dreams from reality<br>• Confused thinking<br>• New academic problems |

*(continued on next page)*

| Table 2 (continued) | |
| --- | --- |
| **Mental Disorder** | **Common Symptoms** |
| | • Extreme moodiness<br>• Personality changes<br>• Ideas that people are out to get them or talking about them (paranoia)<br>• Severe anxiety and fearfulness<br>• Difficulty relating to peers and/or keeping friends<br>• Withdrawal and increased isolation<br>• Worsening personal grooming |

*Data from* American Psychiatric Association. Diagnostic and Statistical Manual of Mental Disorders, 5th Edition: DSM 5. Washington, DC: American Psychiatric Association; 2013.

### Bipolar Disorder

Bipolar disorder, also known as manic-depression, is a mental disorder that is, distinguished by rapid and dramatic changes in mood, affect, and activity. The prevalence of the disorder is equal for men (2.9%) and women (2.8%).[17] Although about 2.8% of adults in the United States have bipolar disorder, about 83% of those have serious impairment.[17] Serious impairment may include physical decompensation from exhaustion and dehydration, serious debt load, and psychosis so sever that suicide occurs. About 3% of adolescents have bipolar disorder with a much smaller rate of impairment.[17] Of course, this statistical is based on those adolescents who reported. The actual prevalence is probably much higher. Common symptoms of manic and depressive symptoms can be seen in **Table 2**.

### SCHIZOPHRENIA

Schizophrenia remains one of the mysteries of mental diseases as well as who is at risk for the disorder. The disorder is one where thought processes are disrupted which cause alterations in perceptions, emotionality, and social relationships. One of the most disabling mental disorders, schizophrenia frequently begins in late adolescence and early adulthood, just as youth may be planning for college or employment. In addition, people with schizophrenia have higher incidence of heart disease, liver disease, and diabetes. Comorbid states may contribute to premature mortality as well as to high suicide rates (4.9%).[18] Schizophrenia is a disease that affects the whole family and community, especially when suicide occurs.[19]

### INTEGRATION OF DEVELOPMENTAL THEORY AND MENTAL HEALTH

Four human development theories and 4 mental disorders were presented for this discussion. So, what does this mean? How are development and behavior connected? If a mental disorder was identified and treated earlier in the lifespan, how would that affect the person and the disease? Would mortality rates decrease? Would there be a decrease in the numbers of people incarcerated?

No matter what developmental theory one might use to guide practice and research, it is clearly important first to know what normal development is. Having that foundation makes it easier to identify abnormal or delayed development. Infant mental health is crucial for lifelong health; when disruptions such as maternal death, sexual abuse, physical abuse, or life threatening illness occur from birth into early childhood, imprints are made on neural pathways that may last a lifetime. One of the reasons the federal

Head Start program was started in 1965 was to provide education for low income children in an effort to mitigate systemic poverty. Poverty is a known risk factor for both poor physical and mental health outcomes and can alter the developmental trajectory. For example, if adequate nutrition is not available because a family cannot afford nutritious food or lives in a food desert, a child's social and school performance can suffer. Undesired behaviors may result which, in turn, affect school attendance as well educational progression. As the school trajectory spirals to expulsion because of brain growth, a child can be well on the way to delinquent behavior and incarceration. Mitigating the previously mentioned cascade has been the intent of both Head Start programs and community programs such as the Nurse-Family Partnership (NFP).[20]

The NFP was created to empower women to have healthy pregnancies, support new mothers to create heathy environments for their infants, and establish trusting relationships with nurses who visited them. The NFP program is guided by the developmental theory of human ecology to affect maternal and child health and child development. Research suggests that the preterm birthrate was significantly lower in the NFP cohort.[21] Beginning a healthy start as an infant can contribute to a normal developmental trajectory as Piaget postulated. Conversely, another study suggests that infants exposed to prenatal maternal substance use and early violence may be at risk for increased violent behavior in early adolescence.[22] Healthy pregnancies, substance use, financial stress are examples of ecological factors that create the epigenetics surrounding an infant. Genetics, prenatal factors, and ecological interactions can contribute to mental health and illness.[23]

Bronfenbrenner described the interactions the infant has with others within the environment as the human developmental trajectory. When the environment is nurturing, present, and healthy, the infant's development can ensue. When the environment is violent, trauma inducing or otherwise harmful, the results of adverse childhood events (ACEs) that occur have longstanding effects on infants and children across the lifespan. For example, ACEs have a strong impact on adolescent health, smoking, obesity, alcohol use, illicit drug use, sexual behavior, and mental health.[24] These behaviors increase the risk of violence and revictimization, relationships, and workforce performance, all affecting the mental health of the human. Furthermore, the impact of the ACEs longtime result is involved with deaths associated with heart disease, diabetes, cancer, and suicide in adults.[25] What is considered normal development for learning and discovering as Piaget postulates is disrupted for the infant, child and youth who experiences maltreatment or who is exposed to toxic stress continuously. The child does not do well in school, may have several DSM 5 diagnoses (if even fortunate enough to have mental health care access), and may start the pathway to delinquency and eventual incarceration. Neurodevelopmental trauma causes chaos, disorganization, and affects physical, cognitive, emotional, and mental spheres. In summary, we know what normal human development is and can be guided by the theories as are described in this paper to assist the growth and development of healthy infants and children.

## IMPLICATIONS FOR NURSING

It is incumbent on us as a caring and knowledgeable discipline with the trust of the public to advocate for early identification and intervention for infants, children, and adolescents. Our social contract with the public requires that we develop evidence-based interventions and conduct research that contributes to our science as well as generate healthy outcomes that increase the quality of life for people. We need to understand that social determinants[26] of communities, policies, and economics can impede mental health. We need to understand that the relationships we have with each other as Bronfenbrenner proposed as the microsystem are the gateways to physically and mentally healthy infants, families, and communities. We need to approach each human through the lens of a biopsychosocial approach as Engel advanced—that a human is more than a disease or the symptoms he presents with or the behaviors that systems find are problematic.

## SUMMARY

Human development is a known entity as many developmental theorists have described. Having a healthful start to life with beneficial prenatal care, wholesome nutrition, adequate and safe shelter sets the stage for subsequent mental health. Although mental illnesses certainly can still occur, a stable environment can promote desired outcomes. Using a developmental approach with people offers a way that looks beyond the behavior or the poverty—it assists us to see the person who is there in all his potential. In this paper, selected developmental theories were presented as well as common mental disorders to provide foundation for understanding how developmental issues interface with mental health.

## REFERENCES

1. Brazelton TB. Touchpoints: birth to 3. Cambridge (MA): Da Capo Press; 2006.
2. Ilg F, Ames LB, Baker SM. Child behavior. New York: Harper Perennial; 1981.
3. Edelman MW. The measure of our success: a letter to my children and yours. Boston: Beacon Press; 1992.
4. Freud S. An outline of psychoanalysis (J. Strachey, Trans.). New York: Norton; 1960.
5. White BL. The first three years of life: the revised edition. New York: Prentice Hall Press; 1985.
6. Crain W. Theories of development: concepts and applications, 4thEd. Upper Saddle River (NJ): Prentice Hall; 2000.
7. Piaget J. Children's understanding of causality. (R.le Cozannet & D. Samson, Trans.). Br J Psychol 1928/2012;18:276–301.
8. Vygotsky LS. The science of psychology. (ME Sharpe, Inc., Trans.). J Russ East Eur Psychol 1928/2012;50(4):85–106.
9. Vygotsky LS. Thought and language. (A. Kozulin, trans.). Cambridge (MA): MIT Press; 1934/1986.
10. Bronfenbrenner U. The ecology of human development. Cambridge (MA): Harvard University Press; 1979.
11. Engel GL. The need for a new medical model: a challenge for biomedicine. Science 1977;196(4286):129–36.
12. Borrell-Carrio F, Suchman AL, Epstein RM. The biopsychosocial model 25 years later: principles, practice, and scientific inquiry. Ann Fam Med 2004;2(6):576–82.
13. Barrane ML, Falissard B. Global burden of mental disorders among children aged 5-14 years. Child Adolesc Psychiatry Ment Health 2018;12:19.
14. National Institute of Mental Health. Depression. National Institute of Mental Health; 2019. Available at: https://www.nimh.nih.gov/health/statistics/major-depression.shtml. Accessed February 17, 2019.
15. American Psychiatric Assosiation. DSM 5. Diagnostic and statistical manual of mental disorders, 5th edition: DSM-5. Washington, DC: American Psychiatric Association; 2013.

16. National Institute of Mental Health. Anxiety. National Institute of Mental Health; 2019. Available at: https://www.nimh.nih.gov/health/statistics/any-anxiety-disorder. shtml. Accessed February 17, 2019.
17. National Institute of Mental Health. Bipolar. National Institute of Mental Health; 2019. Available at: https://www.nimh.nih.gov/health/statistics/bipolar-disorder. shtml. Accessed February 17, 2019.
18. National Institute of Mental Health. Schizophrenia. National Institute of Mental Health; 2019d. Available at: https://www.nimh.nih.gov/health/statistics/schizophrenia.shtml. Accessed February 17, 2019.
19. Powers R. No one cares about crazy people. New York: Hachette Books; 2017.
20. NFP. Nurse Family Partnership. 2019. Available at: https://www.nursefamily partnership.org/about/. Accessed February 17, 2019.
21. Thorland W, Currie DW. Status of birth outcomes in clients of the Nurse-Family Partnership. Matern Child Health J 2017;21(5):995–1001.
22. Terrell S, Conradt E, Dansereau L, et al. A developmental origins perspective on the emergence of violent behavior in males with prenatal substance exposure. Infant Ment Health J 2019;40:54–66.
23. DeSocio JE. Epigenetics, maternal prenatal psychological stress, and infant mental health. Arch Psychiatr Nurs 2018;32(6):901–6.
24. Anda RF, Felitti V, Walker J, et al. The enduring effects of childhood abuse and related experiences: A convergence of evidence from neurobiology and epidemiology. Eur Arch Psychiatry Clin Neurosci 2006;256:174–86.
25. Felitti V, Anda R, Nordenberg D, et al. Relationship of childhood abuse and household dysfunction to many of the leading causes of death: The Adverse Childhood Experiences (ACE) Study. Am J Prev Med 1998;14(4):245–58.
26. World Health Organization (WHO). Closing the gap in a generation: health equity through action on the social determinants of health. Geneva (Switzerland): World Health Organization; 2008.

# Implications of Antipsychotic Use

## Antipsychotic-Induced Movement Disorders, with a Focus on Tardive Dyskinesia

Sattaria Dilks, DNP, PMHNP-BC[a], Rose Mary Xavier, PhD, MS, PMHNP-BC[b],
Crystal Kelly, MSN, FNP[c], Jessica Johnson, PhD, MSN[c],*

## KEYWORDS

- Antipsychotic • Neuroleptic • Dopamine antagonist • Extrapyramidal symptoms
- Movement disorder • Tardive dyskinesia

## KEY POINTS

- Antipsychotics are necessary and life-changing and saving medications, but like all medications they carry the risk of unwanted effects. These effects may include drug-induced movement disorders such as tardive dyskinesia (TD).
- All antipsychotic-treated patients should be screened and monitored for movement disorders. Screening protocols for other antipsychotic-related effects, such as orthostatic hypotension, weight gain, or metabolic changes, already exist.
- Screening may involve a simple visual observation for abnormal movements; however, assessments with formal instruments (eg, Abnormal Involuntary Movement Scale) are recommended.
- Diagnosis of antipsychotic-induced movement disorders are based on the patient's clinical presentation in combination with a thorough psychiatric, medical, and medication history. Differentiating between movement disorders may be challenging, but simple frameworks (eg, acute vs tardive, hypokinetic vs hyperkinetic) can help improve recognition.
- Nurses play a key role in educating patients and families about antipsychotic-induced movement disorders. Central to this education is the availability of FDA-approved medications for TD that allow the patient to remain on their current antipsychotic regimen.

Disclosure Statement: S. Dilks has served as a speaker for Otsuka. R.M. Xavier has served as a consultant to Neurocrine Biosciences, Inc., and has received compensation for this service. C. Kelly and J. Johnson are full-time employees of Neurocrine Biosciences, Inc.
[a] McNeese State University, College of Nursing and Health Professions, 4205 Ryan Street, Lake Charles, LA 70605, USA; [b] The University of North Carolina at Chapel Hill, School of Nursing, Carrington Hall, CB #7460, Chapel Hill, NC 27599-7460, USA; [c] Neurocrine Bioscience, Inc., 12780 El Camino Real, San Diego, CA 92130, USA
* Corresponding author.
*E-mail address:* jjohnson@neurocrine.com
twitter: @rosexavierPhD (R.M.X.)

Nurs Clin N Am 54 (2019) 595–608
https://doi.org/10.1016/j.cnur.2019.08.004      **nursing.theclinics.com**
0029-6465/19/© 2019 The Author(s). Published by Elsevier Inc. This is an open access article under the CC BY-NC-ND license (http://creativecommons.org/licenses/by-nc-nd/4.0/).

## ANTIPSYCHOTIC USE AND DEVELOPMENT

Advancements in the development of antipsychotic medications have led to life-saving outcomes in patients with various psychiatric and nonpsychiatric conditions. Before the introduction of chlorpromazine in psychiatric clinical practice in 1952, there were no effective medications for the treatment of schizophrenia, which is one of the leading causes of disability worldwide.[1,2] The first-generation antipsychotics, also known as "neuroleptics" or "typical" antipsychotics, were primarily dopamine $D_2$ receptor antagonists. These medications continue to be used in schizophrenia and other psychotic disorders because they are effective in managing symptoms such as delusions, hallucinations, and disorganized speech, thoughts, or behavior.

The development of second- and third-generation antipsychotics, also called "atypical" antipsychotics, has resulted in a substantial increase in antipsychotic use.[3] Currently, antipsychotics are routinely prescribed (both on-label and off-label) in numerous psychiatric and neuropsychiatric conditions beyond schizophrenia, including mood and affective disorders, Tourette syndrome, hyperactivity, and challenging behaviors in patients with intellectual developmental disability or other neurodevelopmental disorders (Table 1). Furthermore, use has expanded beyond disorders with psychotic components to conditions such as major depressive disorder, which are often treated in the primary care setting. Newer-generation antipsychotics, including aripiprazole, brexpiprazole, and cariprazine, are partial $D_2$ agonists that act as functional agonists or functional antagonists depending on the surrounding levels of endogenous dopamine (Box 1). When a full agonist is not available, partial agonists bind to the receptors and increase postsynaptic activity (partial agonist); when a full agonist is available, the partial agonist binds to receptors but results in decreased activity compared with full agonist binding (partial antagonist).[4]

Based on their pharmacology, it was believed that the newer antipsychotics would reduce the unwanted effects associated with older antipsychotics, including antipsychotic-induced movement disorders such as tardive dyskinesia (TD), akathisia, dystonia, and parkinsonism. However, the newer medications did not eliminate this risk, as shown in a recent meta-analysis of antipsychotic clinical trials, which estimated the prevalence of TD as 20.7% for second-generation antipsychotics and 30.0% for first-generation antipsychotics.[5] It is worth noting, however, that this meta-analysis also showed that in patients who received second-generation antipsychotics TD prevalence was 7.2%, despite never being exposed to a first-generation antipsychotic.

In this era of increased antipsychotics use, along with the ongoing risk for unwanted movement disorders, all patients should be regularly screened for any sign of abnormal or uncontrollable movements. Drug-induced movement disorders can be highly disruptive, causing behavioral disturbances, exacerbation of psychosis, reduction in quality of life, impairment of working memory performance, and increased treatment nonadherence.[6–9] Furthermore, the failure to diagnose and treat such disorders can lead to significant morbidity or mortality.[10] Therefore, increased awareness is needed about how these disorders present and how they can be treated.

## ANTIPSYCHOTIC-INDUCED MOVEMENT DISORDERS

Historically, antipsychotic-induced movement disorders were called extrapyramidal symptoms (EPS). Because these movement disorders are distinct in presentation and pathophysiology, EPS is obsolete as an umbrella term for all antipsychotic-induced movement disorders. Its use is also clinically problematic because these disorders are not treated in the same way.

**Table 1**
Antipsychotics and indicated uses

| Antipsychotic Generic (Brand) Name | Indicated Use(s) | | | |
| | Schizophrenia or Schizoaffective Disorder | Mood or Other Affective Disorders | Other Psychiatric Disorders | Other Medical Conditions |
|---|---|---|---|---|
| First generation[54,55] | | | | |
| Chlorpromazine (Thorazine)[56] | • Schizophrenia | • Bipolar disorder (manic) | • Hyperactivity (children)<br>• Severe behavioral problems (children) | • Nausea and vomiting<br>• Restlessness and apprehension before surgery<br>• Acute intermittent porphyria<br>• Adjunctive treatment of tetanus<br>• Intractable hiccups |
| Fluphenazine (Prolixin)[57] | | | • Psychotic disorders | |
| Haloperidol (Haldol)[58] | • Schizophrenia | | • Tourette syndrome<br>• Hyperactivity<br>• Severe behavioral problems (children) | |
| Loxapine (Loxitane, Adasuve)[59] | • Schizophrenia | | | |
| Perphenazine (Trilafon)[60] | • Schizophrenia | | | |
| Pimozide (Orap)[61] | | | • Tourette syndrome | |
| Thioridazine (Mellaril)[62] | • Schizophrenia in patients who have failed other antischizophrenia therapy | | | |
| Thiothixene (Navane)[63] | • Schizophrenia | | | |
| Trifluoperazine (Stelazine)[64] | • Schizophrenia | | • Nonpsychotic anxiety (short-term) | |

(continued on next page)

**Table 1**
*(continued)*

| Antipsychotic Generic (Brand) Name | Indicated Use(s) | | | |
|---|---|---|---|---|
| | Schizophrenia or Schizoaffective Disorder | Mood or Other Affective Disorders | Other Psychiatric Disorders | Other Medical Conditions |
| Second and third generation[54,55,65] | | | | |
| Aripiprazole (Abilify)[66] | • Schizophrenia | • Bipolar disorder (manic, mixed)<br>• Adjunctive treatment of major depressive disorder | • Autism<br>• Tourette syndrome | |
| Asenapine (Saphris)[67] | • Schizophrenia | • Bipolar disorder (manic, mixed) | | |
| Brexpiprazole (Rexulti)[68] | • Schizophrenia | • Adjunctive treatment of major depressive disorder | | |
| Cariprazine (Vraylar)[69] | • Schizophrenia | • Bipolar disorder (manic, mixed) | | |
| Clozapine (Clozaril, Verscloz, FazaClo)[70] | • Schizoaffective disorder<br>• Treatment-resistant schizophrenia | | | |
| Iloperidone (Fanapt)[71] | • Schizophrenia | | | |
| Lurasidone (Latuda)[72] | • Schizophrenia | • Bipolar disorder (depressive) | | |
| Olanzapine (Zyprexa)[73] | • Schizophrenia | • Bipolar disorder<br>• Adjunctive treatment of major depressive disorder | | |
| Paliperidone (Invega)[74] | • Schizoaffective disorder<br>• Schizophrenia | | | |
| Quetiapine (Seroquel)[75] | • Schizophrenia | • Bipolar disorder<br>• Adjunctive treatment of major depressive disorder | | |
| Risperidone (Risperdal)[76] | • Schizophrenia | • Bipolar disorder (manic, mixed) | • Autism | |
| Ziprasidone (Geodon)[77] | • Schizophrenia | • Bipolar disorder (manic, mixed) | | |

*Data from Refs.[54–77]*

---

**Box 1**
**Definitions**

*Agonist*: An agonist binds to the receptor and activates it, similar to the endogenous chemical.

*Partial agonist*: A partial agonist binds to the receptor and activates it. It may functionally serve as an agonist or antagonist based on the level of endogenous chemical in the synapse.

*Antagonist*: An antagonist binds to the receptor but does not activate, reducing postsynaptic activity.

*Direct motor pathway*: The direct motor pathway includes synapses in the basal ganglia and cortex, and primarily serves to initiate purposeful movements.

*Indirect motor pathway*: The indirect motor pathway also includes synapses in the basal ganglia and cortex but primarily serves to inhibit unwanted motor contractions.

---

A differential diagnosis of antipsychotic-induced movement disorders can be challenging, but some basic descriptive categorizations (e.g., acute vs tardive, hypokinetic vs hyperkinetic) offer a working framework for recognizing—and appropriately managing—these disorders (**Fig. 1**). Acute syndromes generally present within hours to days of initiating antipsychotic treatment, whereas tardive syndromes are usually associated with more prolonged antipsychotic exposure (months to years). Hypokinetic movement disorders, such as parkinsonism, are characterized by slow or insufficient movements. They are associated with an amplification of the indirect motor pathway, which is mainly responsible for reducing the speed and magnitude of movements.[11] Hyperkinetic movement disorders, such as TD, are characterized by excessive movements. Although not fully understood, it is thought that the pathophysiology of these disorders is primarily associated with dopamine imbalance in the direct motor pathway, which is responsible for increasing the velocity and amplitude of movements. However, hyperkinetic movement disorders may also involve stimulation of $D_2$ receptors in the indirect motor pathway, resulting in decreased activity in this pathway that normally inhibits movement speed and magnitude.

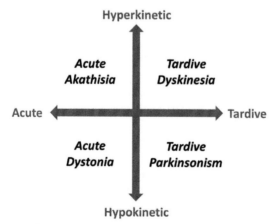

Fig. 1. Differentiation of movement disorders. Examples are provided to show how movement disorders can be differentiated. Of note, however, most abnormal movement types can be "acute" or "tardive" based on when symptoms occur. For example, parkinsonism that appears within a few days or weeks of initiating or changing antipsychotic treatment may be considered "acute."

Four common types of antipsychotic-induced movement disorders are described here and summarized in **Table 2**. This list is intended to be illustrative rather than exhaustive. The purpose is to show that all movement disorders are not the same, describe some of the key differentiating features, and highlight the role that nursing can play in recognizing these disorders.

## Akathisia

Akathisia is a common antipsychotic-induced movement disorder[12,13] characterized by feelings of inner restlessness or tension. Estimates of akathisia prevalence among neuroleptic-treated patients ranges from 18% to 40%, with higher prevalence associated with certain drugs such as haloperidol.[14–18] Patients may indicate an urge to move, are unable to keep still, or exhibit fidgety movements, all of which can be

**Table 2**
**Symptoms and treatment of select antipsychotic-induced movement disorders**

| Movement Disorder | Symptoms | Management or Treatment |
|---|---|---|
| Acute akathisia[20] | • Complaints of restlessness<br>• Excessive fidgety movements (eg, pacing, rocking, inability to sit/stand still)<br>• Symptoms typically develop within a few weeks of starting antipsychotic or raising dose | • Reduce dose or switch antipsychotic<br>• β-Blocker (eg, propranolol) or antihistaminic agent if β-blocker contraindicated (eg, mirtazapine)<br>• Benzodiazepines (eg, clonazepam) |
| Acute dystonia[24] | • Severe muscle spasms of the eyes (oculogyric crisis), head, neck (torticollis), limbs, or trunk<br>• Severe arching of the back or laryngospasm may occur<br>• Symptoms typically emerge within a few days of starting antipsychotic or raising dose | • Reduce dose or switch antipsychotic<br>• Anticholinergics (eg, benztropine)<br>• Antihistaminergic agents (eg, diphenhydramine)<br>• Benzodiazepines<br>• Physical therapy |
| Parkinsonism[26,27] | • Tremor<br>• Muscular rigidity<br>• Akinesia (loss of movement or difficulty initiating movement)<br>• Bradykinesia (slowness of movement)<br>• Symptom onset typically occurs within a few weeks to months of starting antipsychotic or raising dose | • Reduce dose or switch antipsychotic<br>• Anticholinergics<br>• Amantadine |
| Tardive dyskinesia[44] | • Involuntary, hyperkinetic, repetitive choreoathetoid movements<br>• Most commonly observed movements occur in the orofacial region (eg, tongue protruding, facial grimacing, chewing motions of the jaw, excessive blinking)<br>• Movements in extremities/trunk may also occur | • Vesicular monoamine transporter 2 (VMAT2) inhibitors (deutetrabenazine, valbenazine)[a]<br>• Only FDA-approved treatments |

[a] Approved by the United States Food and Drug Administration (FDA).
*Data from* Refs.[13,19,20,22,24,26,34,44,78]

distressing for patients. Most cases will present within 1 to 6 weeks of starting an antipsychotic or increasing an antipsychotic dose.[19] There are no Food and Drug Administration (FDA)-approved treatments specifically for akathisia, although amantadine is approved more generally for drug-induced extrapyramidal reactions in adults. In patients whose psychiatric symptoms will not be exacerbated, the antipsychotic may be switched or the dosage reduced. Though commonly used, there is limited evidence that adjunctive treatment with β-blockers, antihistaminergic agents, or benzodiazepines may alleviate symptoms.[20] Trazodone and mirtazapine (tetracyclic antidepressants) are also used for akathisia.[21,22]

## Acute Dystonia

An estimated 3% to 10% of patients exposed to a neuroleptic agent experience acute dystonia,[23] which is characterized by sustained muscle contractions, abnormal postures, or spasms. Symptoms may present anywhere in the body, with head and neck movements being most common. Symptoms may include back arching, neck extension, or forced eye movements, including oculogyric crisis or the prolonged upward deviation of the eyes. These movements may be dramatic, and patients may be frightened by their appearance. Aside from dystonic laryngospasm, which requires emergency medical intervention, acute dystonia is typically not life threatening. Acute dystonia can occur after a single dose of antipsychotic medication, although most instances emerge over the course of a few days. Treatment may include anticholinergics (eg, benztropine ) or antihistamines (eg, diphenhydramine).[13,19,24] In patients whose psychiatric symptoms will not be exacerbated, the antipsychotic dose may be reduced or the antipsychotic switched.

## Parkinsonism

Antipsychotic-induced parkinsonism (or Parkinson-like symptoms) shares clinical features with Parkinson disease but occurs during antipsychotic use. Recently, a 30-year population-based study found the annual incidence rate of drug-induced parkinsonism to be 3.3 per 100,000 person years, with typical antipsychotics being the most common cause.[25] Symptoms may include bradykinesia, bilateral and symmetric rigidity, postural instability, and tremor. Typical onset is within 1 to 3 months of starting or increasing an antipsychotic dosage. Parkinsonism is best managed by modifying the antipsychotic regimen (ie, tapering and stopping the antipsychotic or switching to another antipsychotic) in patients whose psychiatric disease will not be affected. If the antipsychotic regimen cannot be adjusted, anticholinergics or amantadine may be used instead.[13,19,26,27]

## Tardive Dyskinesia

In a prospective cohort study of outpatients from a community mental health center who received antipsychotics for ≥3 months, 31.5% of evaluated patients had TD on study entry,[28] consistent with the prevalence of 30.0% for first-generation antipsychotics found in the meta-analysis of antipsychotic clinical trials.[5] Among the community outpatients who did not have TD at study entry, the average incidence rate of new TD was 0.066 per patient-year. TD is a persistent and potentially irreversible movement disorder associated with prolonged exposure to antipsychotics. TD is characterized by uncontrollable movements of the head, face, trunk, or limbs,[29–32] and may present as irregular contractions, lip smacking, tongue protrusions, chewing movements of the jaw, facial grimacing, slow writhing in the trunk or extremities, twisting or dance-like movements, and/or tapping of the fingers and toes.[13,33] According to the *Diagnostic and Statistical Manual of Mental Disorders, Fifth Edition* (DSM-5) criteria,[34] a TD diagnosis requires use of an antipsychotic for at least a few months (and possibly shorter in older patients). The DSM-5 also recommends that the movements, if they appear after antipsychotic discontinuation, or change or reduction in dosage, be present for at least 4 to 8 weeks to rule out withdrawal-emergent dyskinesia, which develops after discontinuation or a reduction in dosage of an antipsychotic and typically resolves within 4 to 8 weeks.

The delayed onset of this disorder means that it is often overlooked and underdiagnosed. Furthermore, TD may coexist with other movement disorders, leading to potential misdiagnosis. Patients may also experience considerable physical, social, and functional impacts because of their abnormal movements.[35–38]

Until recently, treatment options for TD were limited to altering the offending antipsychotic, off-label uses of medications (e.g., anticholinergics which can exacerbate TD) and herbal supplements for which evidence was either weak or limited.[39] In 2017, however, a novel vesicular monoamine transporter 2 (VMAT2) inhibitor, valbenazine, was the first medication approved by the FDA for the treatment of adults with TD[40]; deutetrabenazine, a molecular form of tetrabenazine, was approved later that year.[41] Having been evaluated in rigorous double-blind, placebo-controlled clinical trials that demonstrated their efficacy and safety,[42–44] both drugs have shown strong evidence as first-line therapies for TD.[44]

## CLINICAL PRACTICE: A KEY ROLE FOR NURSES

No 2 clinical practices are the same, and the constraints on nurses' time and attention can be considerable. However, there are several specific areas in which nurses play a key role in optimizing care for patients with TD: screening and assessments, education and resources, and treatment support (**Fig. 2**).

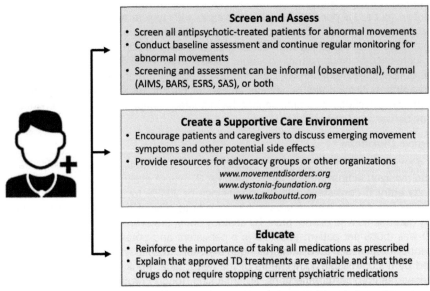

Fig. 2. Nurses' roles in optimizing patient care. AIMS, Abnormal Involuntary Movement Scale; BARS, Barnes Akathisia Rating Scale; ESRS, Extrapyramidal Symptom Rating Scale; SAS, Simpson-Angus Scale.

### Screening and Assessments

Nurses should be aware that all patients taking antipsychotics, especially long term, should be monitored for the development of antipsychotic-induced abnormal movements. Ideally, screening would occur before antipsychotic initiation and any change in therapy (antipsychotic switch or dose increase/decrease), with regular assessments throughout the course of treatment.[33] In many practices, patients are regularly checked for other adverse events associated with antipsychotics (eg, orthostatic hypotension, hyperprolactinemia, weight gain[45]). An assessment of the patient's movements could be incorporated into that protocol.

Screening may be informal, including simple visual observations; regular assessments can be more formal, using validated scales (**Table 3**). These include the Barnes Akathisia Rating Scale[46] for akathisia, the Simpson-Angus Scale[47] for parkinsonism, and the Abnormal Involuntary Movement Scale[48] for TD. The Extrapyramidal Symptom Rating Scale[49] can be used to differentiate between parkinsonism, akathisia, dystonia, and dyskinesia. It should be noted, however, that the diagnostic application of these scales is limited; they are more suited for assessing the severity of abnormal movements and monitoring changes over time. Diagnoses of antipsychotic-induced movement disorders are based on clinical presentation and the patient's psychiatric and medical history, including exposure to antipsychotics or other dopamine-receptor blocking agents such as antiemetics (eg, metoclopramide); a few cases of antidepressant-associated TD have also been reported.[50,51] For TD, the American Psychiatric Association recommends an assessment at antipsychotic initiation and every 3 to 12 months thereafter, with the frequency of assessment depending on the type of antipsychotic used and other risk factors (eg, older age, history of other drug-induced movements).[52] Now that approved TD treatments are available,[42,43] early identification ensures that patients receive timely treatment, which may minimize the negative physical and psychosocial effects associated with TD when left untreated.[35–38]

Not all patients report having abnormal movements, possibly because of underlying diagnosis (eg, schizophrenia versus mood disorder), embarrassment, greater concern about other psychiatric or medical conditions, or lack of knowledge that the movements may be due to their antipsychotic treatment. Some patients with severe schizophrenia may not be aware that they are experiencing movements at all. By contrast, patients with well-controlled mood disorders are more likely to be aware of their movements and highly distressed by even so-called mild irregularities. Given the heterogeneity of the patient population, screening and assessments should be multifaceted and include all patients who receive antipsychotic treatments.[53] Often, caregivers and/or family members are also able to provide information, especially in cases where patients are not aware of their abnormal movements.

### Education, Resources, and Treatment Support

Nurses play a crucial role in building supportive and therapeutically effective relationships with patients and their caregivers. As such, they are uniquely positioned to educate patients regarding the risks for antipsychotic-induced movement disorders. More importantly, they can reassure patients that effective treatments may be available if the appropriate diagnosis is made. In addition, nurses and other health care professionals can point patients to resources such as Web sites that provide support and advocacy for patients and families (see **Fig. 2**; www.movementdisorders.org; www.dystonia-foundation.org; www.talkabouttd.com).

Perhaps the greatest impediment to the discussion of unwanted antipsychotic effects is the fact that the offending medication cannot be eliminated. Patients often

**Table 3**
**Commonly used movement rating scales**

| Rating Scale (Hyperlinked) | Domains or Items | Scoring |
|---|---|---|
| Abnormal Involuntary Movement Scale | • Orofacial movements (4 items)<br>• Movements in trunk or extremities (3 items)<br>• Global judgments (3 items)<br>• Dental status (2 items) | • Items scored on a 5-point scale (0 = none to 4 = severe), with the exception of dental status items, which are yes/no responses<br>• Higher scores (total score is calculated by summing scores from body regions) indicate greater severity of abnormal movements |
| Barnes Akathisia Rating Scale | • Objective measures<br>• Awareness of or distress from restlessness<br>• Global assessment | • First 2 domains scored on a 4-point scale (0 = normal/no distress/absent to 3 = severe/constant movement)<br>• Third domain is rated on a 6-point scale (0 = absent to 5 = severe)<br>• Higher scores indicate greater severity |
| Extrapyramidal Symptom Rating Scale | • Parkinsonism questionnaire<br>• Clinician examination for parkinsonism and akathisia, dystonia, and dyskinesia<br>• Global impression of movement severity | • First domain scored on a 4-point scale (0 = absent to 3 = severe)<br>• Second domain items scored on 7-point scales (0 = absent to 6 = extremely severe)<br>• Third domain scored on a 9-point scale (0 = absent to 8 = extremely severe)<br>• Higher scores indicate greater severity |
| Simpson-Angus Scale | • Assesses changes in the following: gait, arm dropping, shoulder shaking, elbow and wrist rigidity, head rotation, glabella tap, tremor, salivation, and akathisia | • Domains scored on a 5-point scale (0 = absence of condition to 4 = condition present in extreme form)<br>• Total score calculated by summing domain scores and dividing by 10<br>• Higher scores indicate greater severity |

*Data from* Seida J, Schouten J, Mousavi S, et al. First- and second-generation antipsychotics for children and young adults. In: Comparative Effectiveness Reviews No. 39. Rockville, MD: Agency for Healthcare Research and Quality; 2012; and Gervin M, Barnes TRE. Assessment of drug-related movement disorders in schizophrenia. Advances in Psychiatric Treatment. 2000;6:332-341.

require the antipsychotic to maintain psychiatric stability; discontinuing the drug or changing the dose may not be ideal or even feasible. In the case of TD the movements can be irreversible, so changing or discontinuing the dose of the antipsychotic may not resolve the movements. Health care professionals, patients, and caregivers may erroneously believe that the choice is also between treating the psychiatric condition or alleviating the movement disorder. However, in the case of TD, approved medications are available, and these medications have been studied and proved safe to use in conjunction with the patient's stable antipsychotic therapy. Nurses can optimize patient care by reinforcing the importance of taking medications as recommended and referring them to pharmacists or other professionals if specific questions about dosing or drug interactions arise.

## SUMMARY

For many patients, antipsychotics are necessary and potentially life-saving medications; however, they come with certain unavoidable risks, including antipsychotic-induced movement disorders. Nurses play an important role in the recognition, assessment, and management of these antipsychotic-induced movement disorders. In the case of TD, there are now FDA-approved medications that can be taken while continuing with current antipsychotic therapy.

## ACKNOWLEDGMENTS

Medical writing and editorial services were provided by Mary Clare Kane, PhD, and Mildred Bahn, MA, at Prescott Medical Communications Group (Chicago, IL), with support from Neurocrine Biosciences, Inc (San Diego, CA).

## REFERENCES

1. Haddad PM, Correll CU. The acute efficacy of antipsychotics in schizophrenia: a review of recent meta-analyses. Ther Adv Psychopharmacol 2018;8(11):303–18.
2. Lopez-Munoz F, Alamo C, Cuenca E, et al. History of the discovery and clinical introduction of chlorpromazine. Ann Clin Psychiatry 2005;17(3):113–35.
3. Cloud LJ, Zutshi D, Factor SA. Tardive dyskinesia: therapeutic options for an increasingly common disorder. Neurotherapeutics 2014;11(1):166–76.
4. Lieberman JA. Dopamine partial agonists: a new class of antipsychotic. CNS Drugs 2004;18(4):251–67.
5. Carbon M, Hsieh CH, Kane JM, et al. Tardive dyskinesia prevalence in the period of second-generation antipsychotic use: a meta-analysis. J Clin Psychiatry 2017; 78(3):e264–78.
6. Fujimaki K, Morinobu S, Yamashita H, et al. Predictors of quality of life in inpatients with schizophrenia. Psychiatry Res 2012;197(3):199–205.
7. Mathews M, Gratz S, Adetunji B, et al. Antipsychotic-induced movement disorders: evaluation and treatment. Psychiatry 2005;2(3):36–41.
8. Mentzel TQ, Lieverse R, Bloemen O, et al, Genetic Risk and Outcome of Psychosis (GROUP) Investigators. High incidence and prevalence of drug-related movement disorders in young patients with psychotic disorders. J Clin Psychopharmacol 2017;37(2):231–8.
9. Potvin S, Aubin G, Stip E. Antipsychotic-induced parkinsonism is associated with working memory deficits in schizophrenia-spectrum disorders. Eur Arch Psychiatry Clin Neurosci 2015;265(2):147–54.
10. Poston KL, Frucht SJ. Movement disorder emergencies. J Neurol 2008;255(Suppl 4):2–13.
11. Loonen AJ, Ivanova SA. New insights into the mechanism of drug-induced dyskinesia. CNS Spectr 2013;18(1):15–20.
12. Kane JM, Fleischhacker WW, Hansen L, et al. Akathisia: an updated review focusing on second-generation antipsychotics. J Clin Psychiatry 2009;70(5): 627–43.

13. Caroff SN, Campbell EC. Drug-induced extrapyramidal syndromes: implications for contemporary practice. Psychiatr Clin North Am 2016;39(3):391–411.

14. Crawford GB, Agar MM, Quinn SJ, et al. Pharmacovigilance in hospice/palliative care: net effect of haloperidol for delirium. J Palliat Med 2013;16(11):1335–41.

15. Halstead SM, Barnes TR, Speller JC. Akathisia: prevalence and associated dysphoria in an in-patient population with chronic schizophrenia. Br J Psychiatry 1994;164(2):177–83.

16. Janno S, Holi M, Tuisku K, et al. Prevalence of neuroleptic-induced movement disorders in chronic schizophrenia inpatients. Am J Psychiatry 2004;161(1): 160–3.

17. Sachdev P. The epidemiology of drug-induced akathisia: Part II. Chronic, tardive, and withdrawal akathisias. Schizophr Bull 1995;21(3):451–61.

18. Berna F, Misdrahi D, Boyer L, et al. Akathisia: prevalence and risk factors in a community-dwelling sample of patients with schizophrenia. Results from the FACE-SZ dataset. Schizophr Res 2015;169(1–3):255–61.

19. Sachdev PS. Neuroleptic-induced movement disorders: an overview. Psychiatr Clin North Am 2005;28(1):255–74.

20. Pringsheim T, Gardner D, Addington D, et al. The assessment and treatment of antipsychotic-induced akathisia. Can J Psychiatry 2018. https://doi.org/10. 1177/0706743718760288.

21. Forcen F. Akathisia: is restlessness a primary condition or an adverse drug effect? Curr Psychiatry 2015;14(1):14–8.

22. Stroup TS, Gray N. Management of common adverse effects of antipsychotic medications. World Psychiatry 2018;17(3):341–56.

23. Goga JK, Seidel L, Walters JK, et al. Acute laryngeal dystonia associated with aripiprazole. J Clin Psychopharmacol 2012;32(6):837–9.

24. van Harten PN, Hoek HW, Kahn RS. Acute dystonia induced by drug treatment. BMJ 1999;319(7210):623–6.

25. Savica R, Grossardt BR, Bower JH, et al. Incidence and time trends of drug-induced parkinsonism: A 30-year population-based study. Mov Disord 2017; 32(2):227–34.

26. Ward KM, Citrome L. Antipsychotic-related movement disorders: drug-induced parkinsonism vs. tardive dyskinesia-key differences in pathophysiology and clinical management. Neurol Ther 2018;7(2):233–48.

27. Shin HW, Chung SJ. Drug-induced parkinsonism. J Clin Neurol 2012;8(1):15–21.

28. Woods SW, Morgenstern H, Saksa JR, et al. Incidence of tardive dyskinesia with atypical versus conventional antipsychotic medications: a prospective cohort study. J Clin Psychiatry 2010;71(4):463–74.

29. Rana AQ, Chaudry ZM, Blanchet PJ. New and emerging treatments for symptomatic tardive dyskinesia. Drug Des Devel Ther 2013;7:1329–40.

30. Waln O, Jankovic J. An update on tardive dyskinesia: from phenomenology to treatment. Tremor Other Hyperkinet Mov (NY) 2013;3. https://doi.org/10.7916/ D88P5Z71.

31. Caroff SN, Davis VG, Miller DD, et al. Treatment outcomes of patients with tardive dyskinesia and chronic schizophrenia. J Clin Psychiatry 2011;72(3):295–303.

32. Zutshi D, Cloud LJ, Factor SA. Tardive syndromes are rarely reversible after discontinuing dopamine receptor blocking agents: experience from a university-based movement disorder clinic. Tremor Other Hyperkinet Mov (NY) 2014;4:266.

33. Jain R, Correll CU. Tardive dyskinesia: recognition, patient assessment, and differential diagnosis. J Clin Psychiatry 2018;(2). https://doi.org/10.4088/JCP. nu17034ah1c.

34. American Psychiatric Association, DSM-5 Task Force. In: Diagnostic and statistical manual of mental disorders: DSM-5, 5th edition. Washington, DC: American Psychiatric Association; 2013.

35. Strassnig M, Rosenfeld A, Harvey PD. Tardive dyskinesia: motor system impairments, cognition and everyday functioning. CNS Spectr 2018;23(6):370-7.

36. Yassa R, Jones BD. Complications of tardive dyskinesia: a review. Psychosomatics 1985;26:305-13.

37. Browne S, Roe M, Lane A, et al. Quality of life in schizophrenia: relationship to sociodemographic factors, symptomatology and tardive dyskinesia. Acta Psychiatr Scand 1996;94:118-24.

38. Ascher-Svanum H, Zhu B, Faries D, et al. Tardive dyskinesia and the 3-year course of schizophrenia: results from a large, prospective, naturalistic study. J Clin Psychiatry 2008;69:1580-8.

39. Summary of evidence-based guideline for clinicians treatment of tardive syndromes—American Academy of Neurology. 2016. Available at: https://www.aan.com/Guidelines/Home/GetGuidelineContent/613. Accessed November 19, 2018.

40. Neurocrine Biosciences. Valbenazine [prescribing information]. San Diego (CA): Neurocrine Biosciences; 2017.

41. Teva Pharmaceutical Industries. Deutetrabenazine [prescribing information]. Jerusalem (IL): Teva Pharmaceutical Industries, LTD; 2017.

42. Teva Pharmaceutical Industries USA. Austedo [prescribing information]. North Wales (PA): Teva Pharmaceuticals USA, Inc.; 2017.

43. Neurocrine Biosciences. Ingrezza [prescribing information]. San Diego (CA): Neurocrine Biosciences, Inc.; 2017.

44. Bhidayasiri R, Jitkritsadakul O, Friedman JH, et al. Updating the recommendations for treatment of tardive syndromes: a systematic review of new evidence and practical treatment algorithm. J Neurol Sci 2018;389:67-75.

45. De Hert M, Detraux J, van Winkel R, et al. Metabolic and cardiovascular adverse effects associated with antipsychotic drugs. Nat Rev Endocrinol 2011;8(2):114-26.

46. Barnes TR. A rating scale for drug-induced akathisia. Br J Psychiatry 1989;154:672-6.

47. Simpson GM, Angus JW. A rating scale for extrapyramidal side effects. Acta Psychiatr Scand Suppl 1970;212:11-9.

48. Guy W. Abnormal Involuntary Movement Scale (117-AIMS), . ECDEU assessment manual for psychopharmacology. Rockville (MD): National Institute of Mental Health; 1976. p. 534-7.

49. Chouinard G, Ross-Chouinard A, Annable L, et al. Extrapyramidal Symptom Rating Scale. Can J Neurol Sci 1980;7:233.

50. Yilmaz R, Ustun D, Tuncer Uzun S, et al. A probable case of movement disorder (tardive dyskinesia) due to duloxetine treatment. Agri 2018;30(4):199-201.

51. Albayrak Y, Ekinci O. Duloxetine-associated tardive dyskinesia resolved with fluvoxamine: a case report. J Clin Psychopharmacol 2012;32(5):723-4.

52. Lehman AF, Lieberman JA, Dixon LB, et al. Practice guideline for the treatment of patients with schizophrenia, second edition. Am J Psychiatry 2004; 161(2 Suppl):1-56.

53. Daniel SJ, Kannan PP, Malaiappan M, et al. Relationship between awareness of tardive dyskinesia and awareness of illness in schizophrenia. Int J Sci Study 2016;4(7):17-20.

54. Seida J, Schouten J, Mousavi S, et al. First- and second-generation antipsychotics for children and young adults. Comparative Effectiveness Reviews No.

39. 2012. Available at: https://www.ncbi.nlm.nih.gov/books/NBK84635/. Accessed November 5, 2018.

55. Scheer C. Differentiating antipsychotics: an overview of properties impacting drug selection. South Easton (MA): Western Schools SC Publishing; 2016.

56. Chlorpromazine. 2016. Available at: https://www.drugs.com/pro/chlorpromazine.html. Accessed October 30, 2018.

57. Prolixin. 2018. Available at: https://www.drugs.com/pro/prolixin.html. Accessed October 30, 2018.

58. Haloperidol. 2018. Available at: https://www.drugs.com/monograph/haloperidol.html. Accessed October 31, 2018.

59. Galen US. Adasuve [prescribing information]. Souderton (PA): Galen US Inc; 2017.

60. Perphenazine. 2017. Available at: https://www.drugs.com/pro/perphenazine.html. Accessed October 30, 2018.

61. Teva Pharmaceuticals USA. Orap [prescribing information]. Sellersville (PA): Teva Pharmaceuticals USA; 2008.

62. Thioridazine. 2017. Available at: https://www.drugs.com/pro/thioridazine.html. Accessed October 30, 2018.

63. Roerig. Navane [prescribing information]. New York: Roerig, Division of Pfizer, Inc.; 2009.

64. Trifluoperazine tablets. 2018. Available at: https://www.drugs.com/pro/trifluo perazine-tablets.html. Accessed October 30, 2018.

65. OptumRx. Therapeutic class overview: atypical antipsychotics. 2017. Available at: https://www.medicaid.nv.gov/Downloads/provider/Atypical_Antipsychotics_ 2017-0314.pdf. Accessed October 31, 2018.

66. Otsuka America Pharmaceutical. Abilify [prescribing information]. Tokyo: Otsuka America Pharmaceutical Inc; 2016.

67. Allergan USA. Saphris [prescribing information]. Irvine (CA): Allergan USA, Inc; 2017.

68. Otsuka America Pharmaceutical. Rexulti [prescribing information]. Tokyo: Otsuka America Pharmaceutical, Inc.; 2018.

69. Allergan USA. Vraylar [prescribing information]. Madison (NJ): Allergan USA, Inc; 2018.

70. HLS Therapeutics. Clozaril [prescribing information]. Rosemont (PA): HLS Therapeutics, Inc.; 2015.

71. Vanda Pharmaceuticals. Fanapt [prescribing information]. Washington, DC: Vanda Pharmaceuticals Inc; 2017.

72. Sunovion Pharmaceuticals. Latuda [prescribing information]. Marlborough (MA): Sunovion Pharmaceuticals Inc; 2018.

73. Lilly USA. Olanzapine [prescribing information]. Indianapolis (IN): Lilly USA, LLC; 2018.

74. ALZA Corp. Invega [prescribing information]. Vacaville (CA): ALZA Corporation; 2007.

75. AstraZeneca. Seroquel [prescribing information]. Wilmington (DE): AstraZeneca; 2009.

76. Janssen Pharmaceuticals. Risperdal [prescribing information]. Titusville (NJ): Janssen Pharmaceuticals, Inc.; 2007.

77. Roerig. Geodon [prescribing information]. New York: Roerig Division of Pfizer Inc; 2017.

78. Salgado A. Mental health and psychiatric nursing skills: extrapyramidal symptom assessment. Available at: http://ifeet.org/files/24.-Extrapyramidal-symptom-assessment.pdf. Accessed October 30, 2018.

# Understanding Culture in Context

## An Important Next Step for Patient Emotional Well-Being and Nursing

Vicki Hines-Martin, PhD, PMHCNS, RN[a],*,
Shaquita Starks, PhD, RN, APRN, FNP-BC, PMHNP-BC[b],
Carla Hermann, PhD, RN[c], Montray Smith, MSN, MPH, RN, LHRM[d],
Jade Montanez Chatman, BSN, RN[e]

### KEYWORDS

- Culture • Social determinants of health • Emotional well-being

### KEY POINTS

- Social determinants serve as the foundation for cultural expression.
- Social determinants experienced during health-related circumstances can function as barriers or facilitators of cultural expression and impact emotional well-being.
- Nursing as a profession must address culture through the lens of social determinants of health to improve health outcomes and emotional well-being for diverse populations.
- Three areas for growth in nursing to address this perspective are to increase diversity in nursing, strengthen education about social determinants of health, and institutionalize mental health promotion as a strategy to support emotional wellness among diverse populations for all nursing specialties and levels.

Disclosure Statement: The submitted article is an original work not previously submitted for or currently under simultaneous publication consideration. There are no financial conflict of interests to report.

[a] School of Nursing, University of Louisville, Room 4055 Building K, HSC, Louisville, KY 40202, USA; [b] Department of Health Promotion and Disease Prevention, Advanced Practice & Doctoral Studies, College of Nursing, The University of Tennessee, The University of Tennessee Health Sciences Center, 920 Madison Avenue, #534, Memphis, TN 38163, USA; [c] Indiana University Southeast, School of Nursing, 4201 Grant Line Road, New Albany, IN 47150, USA; [d] School of Nursing, University of Louisville, Room 3049, Building K, HSC, 555 South Floyd Street, Louisville, KY 40202, USA; [e] School of Nursing, University of Louisville, Room 4053, Building K, HSC, 555 South Floyd Street, Louisville, KY 40202, USA
* Corresponding author.
*E-mail address:* Vphine01@louisville.edu

Regardless of the setting in which nursing care is provided, one of the important goals for patients and their families is support of health and well-being. Nursing is well-recognized as a profession that focuses on not only physical support but also emotional support during periods of transition and crisis. Many factors influence nursing interventions and patient responses. One of the most important patient-related factors is culture.

## CULTURE DEFINED

The US Department of Health and Human Services Office of Minority Health defines culture as "integrated patterns of human behavior that include the language, thoughts, communications, actions, customs, beliefs, values, and institutions of racial, ethnic, religious, or social groups."[1] Others have defined culture as "the learned and shared beliefs, values, and life ways of a designated or particular group which are generally transmitted inter-generationally and influence one's thinking and action modes."[2] Culture is a complex interaction that is, constantly evolving and is influenced by social, political, historical, and contextual factors.

## CULTURE AND WELL-BEING

The underlying purpose for the development and maintenance of culture by any population is to foster subjective and societal well-being. The Centers for Disease Control and Prevention identifies the following about well-being.

> Well-being is a positive outcome that is, meaningful for people and for many sectors of society, because it tells us that people perceive that their lives are going well. Good living conditions (eg, housing, employment) are fundamental to well-being. Tracking these conditions is important for public policy. However, many indicators that measure living conditions fail to measure what people think and feel about their lives, such as the quality of their relationships, their positive emotions and resilience, the realization of their potential, or their overall satisfaction with life—i.e., their 'well-being.' Well-being generally includes global judgments of life satisfaction and feelings ranging from depression to joy.[3]

According to experts on well-being such as Diener,[4] subjective and societal well-being for any cultural group is founded on its ability to achieve implicit and explicit goals. Cultural groups may be individualistic or collectivistic in their beliefs and, as a result, the goals they pursue reflect those beliefs with aspirations of life satisfaction and affective well-being. Overall, cultural groups generally consider the following: (1) whether others around them believe they are living correctly (according to cultural guidelines), (2) whether they enjoy their lives, and (3) whether others important to them believe they are living well. Well-being can represent the degree to which people in a society are achieving the values they hold dear. Culture involves complex interactions that are constantly evolving and are influenced by the social, political, historical, and contextual environments in which they occur resulting in cultural facilitators or barriers that influence life satisfaction and affective/mental well-being.

## CULTURE AS AN IMPORTANT CONCEPT IN HEALTH AND HEALTH CARE

Health is "a resource that allows people to realize their aspirations, satisfy their needs and to cope with the environment in order to live a long, productive, and fruitful life. Health enables social, economic and personal development fundamental to well-being."[3] Culture in the context of health behavior has been identified as "unique shared values, beliefs, and practices that are directly associated with a health-related behavior, indirectly associated with a behavior, or influence acceptance and adoption of the health education message."[5] The influence of culture on health is substantial. It affects perceptions of health, illness, and death; ideas about causes of disease; methods for promoting health; how illness and pain are experienced and expressed; where and when individuals seek help; and the forms of treatment they prefer.

One important institution that impacts culture and well-being is the health care system. Cultural competence is needed to provide culturally congruent care to individuals and groups with diverse values, beliefs, and behaviors. Culturally competent health care systems work to provide improved health outcomes, foster increased respect and mutual understanding between individuals and their care providers, and increased participation from local communities.[6] Cultural competence is defined as the ability of providers and organizations to effectively deliver health care services that meet the social, cultural, and linguistic needs of patients.[7]

## CULTURE AND CULTURE CARE IN CONTEXT

Although much progress has been made in Western approaches to health care in relation to recognizing the need for cultural awareness, cultural sensitivity, and cultural accommodation in health care delivery, there continues to be room for significant growth in adequately addressing the needs of diverse populations in the areas of service adequacy, health equity, and support of well-being. Freshman[8] identifies "that a broader more inclusive perspective is required to clarify foundational issues, expand understanding and intrinsically incentivize behavior change" among health care providers and health care organizations.

Understanding how individuals and groups enact their beliefs through explicit practices is just the beginning in building cultural competence. Increasingly, research and policy-makers have clearly identified that the social determinants of health (SDH) are the scaffold on which culture is built and therefore serve as a barrier and/or facilitator to cultural expression, even in the area of health care. An inability to adequately address the SDH results in health inequities and negatively impacts well-being among all populations; however, minority and culturally diverse populations are disproportionally affected. Marmot,[9] in his body of research on SDH, identifies that competence in health care with global populations must be grounded in an understanding of the upstream factors, such as economic, social, geopolitical, and resource environments (SDH) of those populations being served in addition to the health beliefs they hold. This perspective is also supported by the World Health Organization and the Centers for Disease Control and Prevention.[10,11]

This article discusses health-related conditions or circumstances that have significance for cultural expression as part of coping and well-being—natural disaster, end of life, and chronic stress and poor mental health. The identified circumstances are discussed through the lens of a SDH context. The importance of cultural diversity within the nursing profession as a support for culture in context are discussed. Last, recommendations for new directions in the profession to better address the complexity of cultural competence in the context of SDH with diverse populations are also presented. **Table 1** provides a summary of key terms and definitions.

## NATURAL DISASTERS

Natural disasters are defined as all types of severe weather that have the potential to pose a significant threat to human health, safety, property, critical infrastructure, and homeland security. These events can include storms, floods, tornadoes, hurricanes, wildfires, earthquakes, tsunamis, or any combination thereof.[12] Disasters are stressful

**Table 1**
**Definition of terms**

| Term | Definition | Example |
|------|-----------|---------|
| Culture | Integrated patterns of human behavior that include the language, thoughts, communications, actions, customs, beliefs, values, and institutions of racial, ethnic, religious, or social groups. The learned and shared beliefs, values, and life ways of a designated or particular group, which are generally transmitted intergenerationally and influence one's thinking and action modes. | May include but not limited to diet, dress, spiritual views, types of rituals related to birth/death, and/or gender roles |
| Well-being (emotional/affective) | A positive outcome that is, meaningful for people and for many sectors of society, because it tells us that people perceive that their lives are going well. Well-being generally includes global judgments of life satisfaction and feelings ranging from depression to joy. Well-being can represent the degree to which people in a society are achieving (or not achieving) the values they hold dear. | Accumulation of experiences that affect an individual's subjective world view. The perception may be affected by acute events (eg, trauma/recovery) or as a result of ongoing experiences (discrimination/equity) |
| Cultural competence | Culturally competent health care systems work to provide improved health outcomes, foster increased respect and mutual understanding between individuals and their care providers, and increased participation from local communities. The ability of providers and organizations to effectively deliver health care services that meet the social, cultural, and linguistic needs of patients. | Systems/providers demonstrate inclusion of the perspectives of diverse populations they serve. This inclusion can be culture specific treatments, representations in the health care setting and ongoing collaboration with the population to identify priorities and strategies for cultural integration into and evaluation of services |
| SDH | The upstream factors such as economic, social, geopolitical and resource environments (SDH) of populations that affect health and health outcomes | Key examples are: Availability of resources to meet daily needs (eg, safe housing, food and water) Access to educational, economic, and job opportunities Social norms and attitudes (eg, discrimination, racism, and distrust of government) Political unrest or oppression Residential segregation Exposure to toxic substances and other physical hazards Public safety (violence) Access to health services |

events not only for individuals who suffer from personal loss, but also for the community as a whole.[13,14] During the past 2 decades, natural disasters have impacted the lives of more than 3 million families worldwide and have had a significant economic impact. The incidence of disasters and human toll has increased over time.[15] Andrews and Boyle[16] identify that cultural influences on individuals and families such as daily roles and dynamics, communication patterns in decision making, nutritional patterns, family and social networks, and religious practices will be disrupted in the short or long term during any disaster. Social determinants such as where a person resides, the region that person is located (developed or developing country), if there have been one or more previous disaster events within the setting, and the resources available to the population will have an impact on the ability to enact cultural norms when dealing with the results of natural disasters. What is also of vital importance is the presence or loss of entities or objects that serve as important symbols within a community after a disaster. These symbols may be religious such as churches, they may be infrastructure such as roads, or they may be the devastation of the environment itself, which results in the loss of important geographically based history for individuals who have experienced the disaster. Change in important symbols can result in psychosocial distress. Therefore, natural disaster resources also need to include psychosocial interventions related to those losses to minimize emotional distress, which is a crucial component of restoring individuals' and communities' well-being and mental health.[17,18] Prior social and geopolitical experiences of those who are affected by disaster are also important to their interpretation and sense of hope as they attempt to recover from the disaster. Experiences of multiple disasters and the degree of recovery and experiences of social exclusion or discrimination are all influential in the response to the current disaster being experienced. Witruk and colleagues,[19] in their study of disaster responses in Java, identified that individuals with an ardent belief in a just world believed that the disasters were due to human behavior, and this belief was an influential factor when dealing with natural disasters.

### Disaster Management and Cultural Impact

According to Beach,[20] disaster management is a system used to organize and manage resources to decrease impact vulnerability. Disaster management contains 5 phases, which are prevention, mitigation, preparedness, response, and recovery. The goal is to reduce the potential loss from disaster events and to ensure that disaster victim have ways to recover.[20,21]

Preparedness consists of individuals, families, and communities anticipating personal needs in the disaster event and strategies to meet those needs that include increasing awareness; obtaining supplies such as food, water, shelter; and health care services.[22] With any population experiencing disaster, it is important for those who are assisting with any of the 5 phases of response to become knowledgeable of the perceptions, appraisal, and understanding of threatening events among the population being served and frame communication using that understanding.

The literature shows that there are several cultural features that impact disaster responses such as the decision to evacuate. A systematic review by Thompson and associates[23] described most common factors associated with the decision to evacuate fell into the following broad categories—*disaster related* (expectations/plan, type of evacuation order, prior experience with disaster), environmental (length of residence in the at risk area, supplies and services availability) individual (age, gender, presence of pets, education) and perceived well-being within SDH (attitudes and treatment of the citizens in the host cities, the presence of borders that are in place [either natural or man-made], perceived safety for those being assisted, the ability to take care of basic family needs [food, shelter, water, health care], climate, and the presence of other cultural groups).

### End-of-Life Care

By 2030, older adults will outnumber children for the first time in the history of the United States.[24] The aging American population will bring a growing demand for care of individuals experiencing life-limiting illness and approaching the end of life. In addition to the rapid growth of the older population, America is becoming considerably more culturally diverse. To provide effective care for individuals as they age and approach the end of life, it is imperative that nurses understand cultural backgrounds and modify care according to cultural needs of patients and families.

Essential to the discussion of cultural considerations of end-of-life care is an understanding of the nuances between palliative care and end-of-life care. The goal of palliative care is to improve the quality of life of patients and their families by providing relief from symptoms and the stress associated with a life-threatening illness.[25] Palliative care focuses on addressing physical, social, mental, and spiritual well-being at any point during a patient's illness. Although palliative care is often viewed as being synonymous with end-of-life care, palliative care is much broader and can be appropriate at any stage of a serious illness.[26] End-of-life care is the care and support provided during the time leading up to and surrounding death and is part of, but not all encompassing, the palliative care trajectory.[27] End-of-life care also focuses on improving quality of life by addressing the holistic needs of a patient and their family, but occurs in a narrower time frame than palliative care.

Whether care is categorized as palliative or end-of-life care, the need to consider cultural beliefs and practices of patients is essential to improve the quality of life of patients and families. Cultural beliefs and practices are extremely important as patients and families encounter suffering and attempt to make meaning of their experiences.

Unfortunately, various cultural beliefs and practices are not well-understood by health providers, including nurses. This is especially true when the clinicians' cultural background differs from the patients' and families'.[28] The inability of nurses to understand how cultural beliefs and practices help patients to make meaning of their illness and suffering may lead to disparities in care and add to the suffering experienced.[29]

There has been an increased focus on improving end-of-life care over the past 20 years. The findings of the SUPPORT study[30] highlighted deficiencies in the health care system to care adequately for patients at the end of life. Since that time, there have been numerous initiatives aimed at improving care for individuals as they near the end of life. However, there still exists a lack of knowledge related to the best models of care and research testing models of culturally appropriate care. Studies have documented disparities in care for underrepresented groups such as lower rates of using hospice care,[31] lower rates of completing advance directives,[32] and higher intensity of care at the end of life. Racial differences in preferences for care, decreased trust of the health care system, and ineffective patient–provider communication may account for the higher intensity level of care that minority individuals at the end of life often receive.[33]

It is imperative that nurses caring for patients at the end of life understand that culture is much broader than race and ethnicity. The delivery of culturally competent care includes recognizing the impact of SDH at end of life. Research is beginning to better identify factors related to emotional well-being in older adults, especially those with life-limiting conditions cross-culturally.[34] Studies with diverse samples are needed to identify factors that can be modified and are related to disparities at the end of life.[35] Current literature does indicate that there are 2 critical areas for providing culturally competent nursing care to patients near the end of life—understanding the patient's view of life and death from a cultural and personal standpoint and the nurse's self-assessment. Acknowledging and developing a basic understanding of end-of-life beliefs of the patients and families themselves to allow sharing from their spiritual and cultural perspective needs to be better integrated into patient assessment during this difficult period in their life course.[36,37] With this critical information, health care providers have indicators of patient priorities, strengths, and needs.

Self-assessment that fosters the nurse's awareness of the impact of their own cultural background, defined broadly, on their views of illness, life, and death is also essential. The need for nurses to understand their own cultural perspectives to equip them to provide culturally appropriate end-of-life care is not a new concept,[38] but it is an often overlooked first step. When self-awareness about one's own culture is lacking, the ability to provide culturally competent care is decreased and may lead to the development of moral distress on the part of the nurse.[39]

Cultural humility is now recognized as an essential component to providing optimal care for patients at the end of life. Cultural humility is "a process of openness, self-awareness, being ego-less and incorporating self-reflection and critique after willingly interacting with diverse individuals" as defined by the *National Consensus Project for Quality Palliative Care*.[40] Asking questions about the importance of religiosity and spirituality, family roles, mistrust of the health care system, and patients' and families' beliefs and desires can inform and improve end-of-life care.[41] Milberg coworkers[42] identified in their study of cross-cultural interaction that health care providers made assumptions about the beliefs of patients from diverse backgrounds and were hesitant to ask for fear of inability to handle the unknown that might be revealed. Use of presence and active listening may elicit more information and build levels of trust that will facilitate the provision of culturally appropriate end-of-life care.[43] Nurses also can facilitate the provision of culturally appropriate care by becoming involved in the creation of policies and other guidelines that reflect the importance of respecting and honoring cultural diversity for patients at the end of life.[44]

### Chronic Stress and Poor Mental Health

Cultural context frames the variety of stressors that individuals may experience and also influences how individuals respond to those stressors.[45] It is widely known that prolonged or chronic stress is injurious to an individual's psychological health.[46] Chronic stress is a precursor for allostatic load or wear and tear of the body that occurs when individuals are exposed to threats, real or perceived, with autonomic physiologic responses that are damaging to the body over time.[47] This wear and tear can impact individuals' mental health and well-being negatively.[47,48] Health care providers need to understand that an individual's appraisal of chronic stressors influences their mental health and well-being through the lens of cultural norms.

Worldwide, individuals' mental health and well-being are shaped by their environment, which is primarily influenced by culture and within-culture variances. Cultural dynamics can facilitate or impede individuals' classification of mental illness within their defined groups and can also influence specific groups' consumption and acceptance of mental health services. Culture influences reaction to stressors as well as individuals' health care practices, and beliefs. Chronic stress can impact individuals' mental health and well-being and may differ between and within various cultures.[49]

Gender roles within one's culture may influence chronic stress exposure and the outcome of this exposure over time. For example, women assume responsibility for the many household activities and are responsible for complex and time-consuming caregiving tasks that potentially result in self-care neglect, isolation, anxiety, depression, and resentment.[50,51] In contrast, some cultures are constructed whereby women take pride in providing care to their loved ones and do not view caregiving as a stressor, but as a protective and supportive role.[52,53] Nurses should assess this area because it may be viewed as a potential chronic stressor resulting in poor mental health and well-being.[50,52,54]

There are gender differences in help-seeking behaviors, such as men's adherence to traditional male gender roles that reinforce the perception that help-seeking demonstrates weakness. For instance, among many Latinos, *Machismo*, a traditional male gender role may, prevent them from seeking care for mental health problems because it is considered a threat to their masculinity.[55]

## CULTURE, POLITICAL OPPRESSION, AND MENTAL HEALTH AND WELL-BEING

Refugees who have relocated in the United States often present to health care providers with chronic stress and untreated mental health issues. Many refugees have resettled in the United States because of political oppression and conflict, and present to health care providers with not only physical remnants of trauma and torture but also mental health conditions, primarily posttraumatic stress disorder and depression.[49,56,57] Many providers feel uncomfortable about discussing past trauma for fear or retraumatizing the patient, lack of culturally appropriate tools to start conversations, and inadequate time to explore patient issues.

Time is viewed differently in many cultures; thus, individuals who perceive that health care providers do not have time to talk to them may withhold vital information that is, important to the treatment regimen.[49,58] To establish trust and provide comfort to persons born outside the United States, it is important for health care providers to provide ample time for encounters, inquire about individuals' lives in their country of origin, and listen without interruption.[49]

Inquiring about the historical context of symptoms is an important task when assessing for mental health concerns in foreign born persons. Understanding symptoms in the context in which those problems first occurred is critical, such as symptoms related to war, violence, displacement, and traumatic loss.

## CULTURE-SPECIFIC TRAUMA AND STRUCTURAL RACISM

Nurses must take into consideration the political underpinnings of historical trauma in specific populations such as American Indians who, because of colonialism, continue to experience poor mental health.[59] When nurses fail to acknowledge or believe, or even deny the full scope of trauma experienced by these individuals, it can further damage them. Although the brutal force of colonialism seems to have dissipated, the aftermath of colonialism continues in the form of institutionalized poverty and racism.[60]

The US culture supports social policies that influence stress among African Americans and contribute to the vast disparities in health experienced among this group. Nationally and globally, a measure of a population's health is its infant mortality rate.[61] African American women have the highest infant mortality rates in the United States,[62] despite receiving early and regular prenatal care, higher educational attainment, and income.[63] Chronic stress from a lifetime of structural racism and racial inequity influences health disparities in African American women and their birth outcomes.[64]

Structural racism is described as a system of institutional practices, cultural representations, and public policies that perpetuate racial inequality. The criminal justice system is maintained by these policies and practices that expose African American women to high levels of stress and health disparities.[65,66] Higher rates of incarceration for African American women and the indirect impact on their families dramatically influences the mental health and well-being of children, affecting behavioral, emotional, and developmental adjustment well into adulthood. Additionally, contact with the criminal justice system increases the occurrence of family separation, which ultimately impacts the groups' mental health and well-being.[65]

## HEALTH CARE CULTURE, MENTAL HEALTH, AND WELL-BEING

Nurses and other health care providers should avoid impelling care that excludes the possibility of an individuals' traditional healing practices to strictly adhere to evidence-based guidelines. The current approach to mental health is colonizing, basing diagnosis on customary Western methods of diagnosis, and allowing health care providers to ignore the underlying sources of chronic stressors (ie, racism, discrimination) or trauma that could be triggering certain poor mental presentations. Discounting traditional methods because of the lack of evidence-based data marginalizes honored and traditional ways of healing.[59] Prussing and colleagues[60] reported that use of evidence-based medicine causes health care providers to overlook the social and cultural influences of psychological experiences and important political-economic factors that impact individuals' mental health and well-being.

## ENVIRONMENT, STRUCTURAL FACTORS, AND MENTAL HEALTH AND WELL-BEING

Some individuals flee from their countries of origin for religious, political, or economic reasons. However, they may experience chronic stress as a result of a change in their social environment.[67,68] Place matters as it relates to mental health and well-being.[69] Being culturally embedded in the broader US context where racism, social exclusion, and prejudice prevail is a precursor to chronic stress that negatively impacts mental health. Pina-Watson and associates[70] found that Mexican descent youth experience bicultural stress (eg, identifying with 2 cultures simultaneously), which is associated with poor mental health outcomes. Factors related to bicultural stress (eg, discrimination and language stress) may be unavoidable, and if unaddressed in a therapeutic way, may lead to helplessness when individuals must decide which cultural beliefs, behaviors, and values to adopt from the mainstream culture, and what to retain from their heritage culture.[69]

Many people from ethnic minority groups are more family focused and promote interdependence and cooperative efforts within the family. This cultural factor influences help-seeking behaviors in many Latino families is *Familismo,* or a belief in strong family unity and connection. Because of *Familismo*, persons with depression may seek help from first their family members or spiritual leaders rather than professionals. Latino immigrants may not readily volunteer their feelings about depression to health care providers. Therefore, health care providers should begin exploring this possibility by addressing possible immigrant stress through the lens of its impact on the family and family functioning (ie, experiences of prejudice, adapting to a new environment, and having children reared in a foreign culture), because some patients may not perceive themselves as being depressed, although they will talk about stressful life events.[55]

## *Meeting the Challenge of Culture in Context Within the Nursing Profession*

This article has identified the complexity of culture; the influence of social determinants on the expression of culture; the impact of specific social, political, and environmental factors on cultural enactment; and some ways the interaction between culture and social determinants can affect emotional well-being during critical transitions and periods of crisis. As the growing body of interdisciplinary literature identifies, these interactions have a significant impact on how nurses and other health care professionals should and can function in a variety of settings to address health needs and support affective well-being and mental health. However, there is much work that needs to be done in 3 critical areas to meet the challenge. These are (1) to increase the numbers of nurses from diverse cultural and ethnic backgrounds, (2) strengthen education about SDH across all levels of nursing education and (3) institutionalize the expectation that care targeting affective wellness is a critical aspect of all nursing specialties and levels of care. The following are recommendation related to these 3 important areas.

According to the US Census Bureau,[71] by 2043 the combined racial-ethnic minority populations in the United States will outnumber non-Hispanic whites. Because our population is becoming increasingly diverse, it is crucial that health care workers reflect this diversity and be culturally competent to address health disparities. Registered nurses account for the largest body of health care workers in the United States.[72] According to the American Association of Colleges of Nursing, "nurses from minority backgrounds represent 19% of the registered nurse work force."[73] Because of their numbers, the profession of nursing can have an impact on health outcomes, and health care services, and representation of the diversity of the populations they serve is of critical importance. The National Advisory Council on Nurse Education and Practice supports the recommendation to increase diversity to "improve standards of practice, patient outcomes, and access to care."[74] *The Future of Nursing: Leading Change* document recommends greater emphasis on cultural change in health professions education and increased diversity as priorities for the nursing workforce.[75,76]

Health and wellness are greatly influenced by the SDH, which includes an array of life conditions that have the potential to create chronic stress. Nursing education and health care leadership have identified that future nurses will need skills in addressing the SDH, and delivering health care within the context of the social environment.[77-81] **Fig. 1** proposes a framework for nursing care that incorporates the perspectives that have been presented.

## Nursing in a Person-Centered/Context Driven Model

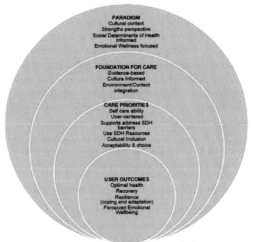

**Fig. 1.** Recommendations for nursing care using culture in context framework. (*Data from* Bronfenbrenner U. The Ecology of Human Development. Cambridge, MA: Harvard University Press; 1979 and Bronfenbrenner U. Toward an experimental ecology of human development. American Psychologist. 1977;32(7): 513-531.)

The *Future of Nursing* report represents an opportunity for nurses in health care delivery. However, to realize a vision that explicitly emphasizes the contribution that nurses can and do make in support of emotional well-being, nurses are challenged to develop a universal understanding and paradigm that focuses on mental health promotion in nursing practice to support emotional wellness in all specialties. As early as 1998, the relationship between emotional well-being and physical health outcomes has been discussed in the literature.[82] However, other health professions[83,84] are steering the conversation. Leading requires raising our voices and presenting clinical exemplars and research in this important area of health.

## REFERENCES

1. U.S. Department of Health and Human Services Office of Minority Health. Assuring cultural competence in health care: recommendations for National standards and outcomes-focused research Agenda. Washington, DC: U.S. Government Printing Office; 2000.
2. Leininger MM. Transcultural care diversity and universality: a theory of nursing. Nurs Health Care 1985;6:208–12.
3. Centers for Disease Control and prevention. Health-Related Quality of Life (HRQOL). Available at: https://www.cdc.gov/hrqol/wellbeing.htm. Accessed December 20, 2018.
4. Diener E, editor. Culture and well-being: the collected works of Ed Diener, social indicators research Series 38. Berlin/Heidelberg (Germany): Springer Science+Business Media B.V; 2009. https://doi.org/10.1007/978-90-481-2352-0_03.
5. Pasick RJ, D'Onofrio CN, Otero-Sabogal R. Similarities and differences across cultures: questions to inform a third generation for health promotion research. Health Educ Q 1994;23(suppl):S142–61.
6. Health Research & Educational Trust. Becoming a culturally competent health care organization. Chicago (IL): Health Research & Educational Trust; 2013. Available at: http://www.hpoe.org. Accessed December 21, 2018.
7. Betancourt JR, Green AR, Carrillo JE. Cultural competence in health care: emerging frameworks and practical approaches. New York: The Commonwealth Fund; 2002.
8. Freshman B. Cultural Competency- Best intentions are not good enough. Divers Equal Health Care 2016;13(3):240–4.
9. Marmot M. Closing the Gap in a generation. World Congress of Epidemiology, Paolo Alegre, Brazil 2008. Available at: http://www.epi2008.com.br/apresentacoes/CONFERENCIA%2023_09_11h45_pdf/Michael%20Marmot.pdf. Accessed December 22, 2018.
10. World Health Organization. About Social determinants of Health. Available at: https://www.who.int/social_determinants/sdh_definition/en/. Accessed December 22, 2018.
11. Centers for Disease Control and Prevention. Social determinants of health: know what affects health 2018. Available at: https://www.cdc.gov/socialdeterminants/. Accessed December 22, 2018.
12. Department of Homeland Security. Natural Disasters 2018. Available at: https://www.dhs.gov/naturaldisasters/. Accessed December 20, 2018.
13. Khankeh HR, Khorasani-Zavareh D, Johanson E, et al. Disaster health-related challenges and requirements: a grounded theory study in Iran. Prehosp Disaster Med 2011;26(3):151–8.

14. Norris FH, Perilla JL, Riad JK, et al. Stability and change in stress, resources, and psychological distress following natural disaster: findings from hurricane Andrew. Anxiety Stress Coping 1999;12(4):363–96.
15. McFarlane AC, Williams R. Mental health services required after disasters: learning from the lasting effects of disasters. Depress Res Treat 2012;2012:970194.
16. Andrews M, Boyle J. Transcultural concepts in nursing care. 5th edition. Dordrecht (Netherlands): Wolters Kluwer; 2008.
17. Burke S. A response by the Australian psychological society to the draft report of the productivity commission inquiry into natural disaster funding 2014. Australian Psychological Society. Available at: https://www.psychology.org.au/Assets/Files/APS%20Response%20to%20Draft%20Productivity%20Commission%20report%20on%20natural%20disaster%20funding.pdf. Accessed December 12, 2018.
18. Reser J, Morrissey S. The crucial role of psychological preparedness for disasters. InPsych: The Bulletin of the Australian Psychological Society 2009;31(2):14–5.
19. Witruk E, Lee Y, Otto K. Dealing with earthquake disaster on Java 2006: a comparison of affected and non-affected people. Anima-Indonesian Psychological Journal 2014;29(3):121–35.
20. Beach M. Disaster preparedness and management. Philadelphia: F.A. Davis; 2010.
21. Federal Emergency Management Agency. Disaster Management Cycle 2018. Available at: https://www.fema.gov/disastermanagement cycle/. Accessed December 20, 2018.
22. Baker L, Cormier L. Disasters and vulnerable populations: evidence-based practice for the helping professions. New York: Springer Publishing Company; 2015.
23. Thompson R, Garfin D, Silver R. Evacuation from natural disasters: a systematic review of the literature. Risk Anal 2017;37(4):812–39.
24. United States Census Bureau. Population projections. Available at: https://www.census.gov/newsroom/press-releases/2018/cb18-41-population-projections.html. Accessed December 21, 2018.
25. World Health Organization. Palliative care. Available at: https://www.who.int/cancer/palliative/definition/en. Accessed December 21, 2018.
26. Center to Advance Palliative Care. Palliative care. Available at: https://www.capc.org/about/palliative-care/. Accessed December 21, 2018.
27. National Institute on Aging. What is end of life care?. Available at: https://www.nia.nih.gov/health/what-end-life-care. Accessed December 21, 2018.
28. Periyakoil VS, Neri E, Kraemer H. Patient-reported barriers to high-quality end-of-life care: a multiethnic, multilingual, mixed-methods study. J Palliat Med 2016;19(4):373–9.
29. Worster B, Bell DK, Roy V, et al. Race as a predictor of palliative care referral time, hospice utilization, and hospital length of stay: a retrospective noncomparative analysis. Am J Hosp Palliat Care 2017;35(1):110–6.
30. SUPPORT Principal Investigators. A controlled trial to improve care for seriously ill hospitalized patients. The study to understand prognoses and preferences for outcomes and risks of treatment (SUPPORT). J Am Med Assoc 1995;274:1591–8.
31. Frahm KA, Brown LM, Hyer K. Racial disparities in end-of-life planning and services for deceased nursing home residents. J Am Med Dir Assoc 2012;13(9):819.e7-11.
32. Frahm KA, Brown LM, Hyer K. Racial disparities in receipt of hospice services among nursing home residents. Am J Hosp Palliat Care 2015;32(2):233–7.
33. Brown CE, Engleberg RA, Sharma R, et al. Race/ethnicity, socioeconomic status, and healthcare intensity at the end of life. J Palliat Med 2018;21(9):1308–16.

34. Steptoe A, Denton A, Stone A. Psychological wellbeing health and ageing. Lancet 2015;385(9968):640–8.

35. Rahemi Z, Williams CL. Older adults of underrepresented populations and their end-of-life preferences an integrative review. ANS Adv Nurs Sci 2016;39(4):E1–29.

36. Fang ML, Sixsmith J, Horst G. A knowledge synthesis of culturally- and spiritually-sensitive end-of-life care: findings from a scoping review. BMC Geriatr 2016;16:107.

37. Gire J. How death imitates life: cultural influences on conceptions of death and dying. Online Readings in Psychology and Culture 2014;6(2). https://doi.org/10. 9707/2307-0919.1120.

38. Matzo ML, Sherman DW, Mazanec P, et al. Teaching cultural considerations at the end of life: end of life nursing education consortium program recommendations. J Contin Educ Nurs 2002;33(6):270–8.

39. Rising ML. Truth telling as an element of culturally competent care at end of life. J Transcult Nurs 2017;28(1):48–55.

40. National Consensus Project for Quality Palliative Care. National Coalition for Hospice and Palliative Care. Available at: https://www.nationalcoalitionhpc.org/ncp/. Accessed December 21, 2018.

41. Cain CL, Surbone A, Elk R, et al. Culture and palliative care: preferences, communication, meaning, and mutual decision making. J Pain Symptom Manage 2018;55(5):1408–19.

42. Milberg A, Torres S, Agard P. Health Care Professional's understanding of cross-cultural interaction in end of life care: a focus group study. PLoS One 2016. https://doi.org/10.1371/journal.pone.0165452.

43. Mazanec P, Burke JT. Cultural considerations in palliative care. In: Ferrell BR, Coyle N, Paice J, editors. Oxford textbook of palliative nursing. 4th edition. Oxford (England): Oxford University Press; 2015. p. 469–82.

44. Bloomer MJ, Botti M, Runacres F, et al. Cultural considerations at end of life in a geriatric inpatient rehabilitation setting. Collegian 2018. https://doi.org/10.1016/j. colegn.2018.07.004.

45. Aldwin CM. Culture, coping and resilience to stress. Proceedings of the First International Seminar on Operationalization of Gross National Happiness. Thimpu, Bhutan: Center for Bhutan studies, February 18-20, 2004.

46. American Psychological Association. Understanding chronic stress. 2018. Available at: https://www.apa.org/helpcenter/understanding-chronic-stress.aspx.

47. Juster RP, McEwen BS, Lupien SJ. Allostatic load biomarkers of chronic stress and impact on health and cognition. Neurosci Biobehav Rev 2010;35(1):2–16.

48. Beckie TM. A systematic review of allostatic load, health, and health disparities. Biol Res Nurs 2012;14(4):311–46.

49. Shannon PJ. Refugees' advice to physicians: how to ask about mental health. Fam Pract 2014;31(4):462–6.

50. Office of Women's Health. Caregiver stress. 2018. Available at: https://www. womenshealth.gov/a-z-topics/caregiver-stress.

51. Okihiro M, Duke L, Goebert D, et al. Promoting optimal native outcomes (PONO) by understanding women's stress experiences. J Prim Prev 2017;38(1–2): 159–73.

52. Campos B, Ullman JB, Aguilera A, et al. Familism and psychological health: the intervening role of closeness and social support. Cultur Divers Ethnic Minor Psychol 2014;20(2):191–201.

53. Starks SA, Outlaw F, Graff JC, et al. Quality of life and African American women who are family caregivers: a literature review with implications for psychiatric

mental health advanced practice registered nurses. Issues Ment Health Nurs 2018;39(6):467–81.

54. Rozario PA, DeRienzis D. Familism beliefs and psychological distress among African American women caregivers. Gerontologist 2008;48(6):772–80.

55. Caplan S, Buyske S. Depression, help-seeking and self-recognition of depression among Dominican, Ecuadorian and Colombian immigrant primary care patients in the northeastern United States. Int J Environ Res Public Health 2015;12(9): 10450–74.

56. Perreira KM, Ornelas I. Painful passages: traumatic experiences and post-traumatic stress among immigrant Latino adolescents and their primary care-givers. Int Migr Rev 2013;47(4):976–1005.

57. Perreira KM, Gotman N, Isasi CR, et al. Mental health and exposure to the United States: key correlates from the Hispanic community health study of Latinos. J Nerv Ment Dis 2015;203(9):670–8.

58. Ge G, Burke N, Somkin CP, et al. Considering culture in physician-patient communication during colorectal cancer screening. Qual Health Res 2009; 19(6):778–89.

59. Keyes J. Decolonizing the mental health system, Hearthside Healing (Blog) 2017. Available at: https://www.hearthsidehealing.com/decolonizing-the-mental-health-system/.

60. Prussing E. Historical trauma: politics of a conceptual framework. Transcult Psychiatry 2014;51(3):436–58.

61. Centers for Disease Control and Prevention. Public health approaches to reducing U.S. infant mortality. 2018. Available at: https://www.cdc.gov/grand-rounds/pp/2012/20121016-infant-mortality.html.

62. Centers for Disease Control and Prevention. Infant mortality. 2018. Available at: https://www.cdc.gov/reproductivehealth/MaternalInfantHealth/InfantMortality.htm.

63. Smith IZ, Bentley-Edwards KL, El-Amin S, et al. Fighting at birth: eradicating the black-white infant mortality gap. Durham (NC): Duke University's Samuel DuBois Cook Center on Social Equity and Insight Center for Community Economic Development; 2018.

64. Center for American Progress. Mass incarceration, stress, and black infant mortality: a case in structural racism. 2018. Available at: https://www.americanprogress.org/issues/race/reports/2018/06/05/451647/mass-incarceration-stress-black-infant-mortality/.

65. National Association for the Advancement of Colored People. Incarceration trends in America. 2018. Available at: https://www.naacp.org/criminal-justice-fact-sheet/.

66. Lee J. Maternal stress, well-being, and impaired sleep in mothers of children with developmental disabilities: a literature review. Res Dev Disabil 2013;34(11): 4255–73.

67. Kizilhan JI. Trauma and pain in family-orientated societies. Int J Environ Res Public Health 2017;15(1) [pii:E44].

68. Stacciarini JM, Smith R, Garvan CW, et al. Rural Latinos' mental wellbeing: a mixed-methods pilot study of family, environment and social isolation factors. Community Ment Health J 2015;51(4):404–13.

69. Weir K. Exploring how location affects mental health. Washington, DC: American Psychological Association; 2017. p. 18.

70. Pina-Watson B, Llamas JD, Stevens AK. Attempting to successfully straddle the cultural divide: hopelessness model of bicultural stress, mental health, and

caregiver connection for Mexican descent adolescents. J Couns Psychol 2015; 62(4):670–81.

71. U.S. Census Bureau. U.S. Census Bureau projections show a slower growing, older, more diverse nation a half century from now. 2012. Available at: https://www.census.gov/newsroom/releases/archives/population/cb12-243.html.

72. Loftin C, Newman SD, Gilden G, et al. Moving toward greater diversity: a review of interventions to increase diversity in nursing education. J Transcult Nurs 2013; 24(4):387–96.

73. American Association of Colleges of Nursing. Fact sheet: enhancing diversity in the nursing workforce. 2015. Available at: www.aacn.nche.edu/media-relations/diversityFS.pdf.

74. National Advisory Council on Nurse Education and Practice (2013). Achieving health equity through nursing workforce diversity: eleventh report to the Secretary of the Department of Health and Human Services and the Congress. U.S. Department of Health and Human Services, Health Resources and Services Administration: Washington, DC. Available at: https://www.hrsa.gov/advisorycommittees/bhpradvisory/nacnep/Reports/eleventhreport.pdf. Accessed 2018.

75. Shalala D, Bolton LB, Bleich MR, et al. The future of nursing: leading change, advancing health. Washington, DC: The National Academies Press; 2011.

76. Smedley BD, Butler AS, Bristow LR. In the Nation's compelling interest: ensuring diversity in the health care workforce. Washington, DC: The National Academies Press; 2004.

77. Advisory Committee on Interdisciplinary, Community-Based Linkages. Transforming interprofessional health education and practice: moving learners from the campus to the community to improve population health. Thirteenth Annual Report to the Secretary of the United States Department of Health and Human Services and the Congress of the United States, October 2014. Rockville, MD: U.S. Department of Health and Human Services, Health Resources and Services Administration. Available at https://www.hrsa.gov/advisorycommittees/bhpradvisory/acicbl/Reports/thirteenthreport.pdf. Accessed December 30, 2018.

78. National Advisory Council on Nurse Education and Practice. Preparing nurses for new roles in population health management. Based on the 132nd and 133rd Meetings of the NACNEP 2016, Health Resources and Services Administration. Rockville (MD), January 12-13, 2016 and June 7-8, 2016.

79. Salmond S, Ecchevarria M. Healthcare transformation and changing roles for nursing. Orthop Nurs 2017;36(1):12–25.

80. Williams SD, Hansen K, Smithey M, et al. Using social determinants of health to link health workforce diversity, care quality and access, and health disparities to achieve health equity in nursing. Public Health Rep 2014;129(Suppl 2):32–6.

81. Lipstein SH, Kellerman AL, Berkowitz B, et al. Workforce for 21st century health and health care series: a vital direction for health and health care. Washington, DC: National Academy of Medicine; 2016.

82. Stewart-Brown S. Emotional wellbeing and its relation to health. BMJ 1998; 317(7173):1608–909.

83. Feller SC, Castillo EG, Greenberg JM, et al. Emotional wellbeing and public health: proposal for a model national initiative. Public Health Rep 2014; 129(Suppl 2):32–6.

84. Coverdale G, Long AF. Emotional wellbeing and mental health: an exploration into health promotion in young people and families. Perspect Public Health 2015. https://doi.org/10.1177/1757913914558080.

# Compassion Fatigue in Advanced Practice Registered Nurses
## Why Don't We Know More?

Lindsay Bouchard, DNP, PMHNP-BC, RN

## KEYWORDS

- Professional quality of life • Compassion fatigue • Burnout
- Secondary traumatic stress • Advanced practice registered nurse
- Nurse practitioner

## KEY POINTS

- Compassion fatigue (CF) can negatively affect health care professionals' mental and physical health, productivity, and quality of patient care.
- Advanced practice registered nurses (APRNs) may be at high risk for developing CF due to their work environments, engagement in patient care, and personal attributes.
- Both individual and organizational actions can mitigate CF.
- Additional research is needed to explore how APRNs develop, experience, and alleviate CF.

## INTRODUCTION

Advanced practice registered nurses (APRNs) are a growing part of the health care workforce. In the United States, there are now more than 248,000 licensed APRNs with more than 26,000 graduating within the last 2 years.[1] Understanding how to improve professional quality of life for APRNs is critical for an efficient health care system that best promotes patients' wellbeing. Health care providers' aggregate work stress and the resulting emotional, social, and physical toll and deleterious impact on their patient care are well documented in the literature.[2–4] Enhancing the work life of health care providers is imperative to improving patient outcomes and has been suggested as a "Quadruple Aim" essential to accomplishing the Institute for Healthcare Improvement "Triple Aim" framework for optimizing the performance of

Disclosure Statement: Dr L. Bouchard has no commercial or financial conflicts of interest or funding sources to disclose.
College of Nursing, University of Arizona, 1305 North Martin Avenue, Tucson, AZ 85721, USA
*E-mail address:* labouchard@email.arizona.edu

Nurs Clin N Am 54 (2019) 625–637
https://doi.org/10.1016/j.cnur.2019.08.002
0029-6465/19/© 2019 Elsevier Inc. All rights reserved.

our health care system (improving population health, reducing health care costs, and ameliorating the patient care experience).[2,5,6] A large threat to professional quality of life is compassion fatigue (CF), which can negatively affect health care professionals' mental and physical health, productivity, and quality of patient care. CF is commonly conceptualized as the combined negative effects of burnout and secondary traumatic stress and may be offset by positive compassion satisfaction (CS).[7,8] Research conducted with a variety of health care professionals indicates that APRNs' work responsibilities, patient care, and personal attributes may place them at high risk for developing CF. Despite the current paucity of published research regarding how APRNs develop and experience CF, APRNs should be aware of the potential causes, symptoms, and negative effects of this phenomenon due to its impact on health care providers, patients, and organizations. Documented symptoms of CF for health care professionals include multiple detrimental emotional, physical, and behavioral changes that can deteriorate the quality of patient care.[2,3,9] Behaviors associated with CF such as substance abuse,[10] poor clinical judgment,[2] higher rates of medical errors,[9] and increased medical lawsuits[9] may also jeopardize the ability to maintain professional licensure. Burnout in APRNs is associated with hospital-acquired infections in low-weight neonates,[11] poor culture of safety scores,[9] and turnover.[12–14] This review discusses CF in APRNs, including the contributing factors, potential interventions, and suggested avenues for future research.

## DISCUSSION

Since CF's appearance in the literature in the early 1990s,[15,16] there has been a growing body of research related to its effects. CF can affect a variety of professionals; in 2018 alone, published research addressed the phenomenon of CF or burnout in many non–health care–related professions, such as educators,[17,18] school counselors,[19] police officers,[20] social workers,[21] clergy,[22] managers,[23] farmers,[24] therapists,[25] animal care professionals,[26,27] athletes,[28] firefighters,[29] massage therapists,[30] and adult and child protective services workers.[31,32] Within the health care field, studies regarding CF include samples of medical and nursing students,[33–35] pharmacists,[36] prehospital personnel,[37,38] professional caregivers,[39] mental health professionals,[40,41] genetic counselors,[42] occupational therapists,[43] nursing faculty,[44] nurses working in a variety of settings,[2,45] physician assistants (PAs),[46,47] and physicians of different specialties[2,3]; however, there is limited published research that includes APRNs.

### The Concept of Compassion Fatigue

Broadly, CF is the result of the stress of caring for others who are physically or mentally suffering.[48] Reported potential symptoms of CF are physical, behavioral, psychological, and spiritual[2–4,7,9] (**Box 1**). Risk factors are thought to include intense and prolonged contact with patients, the use of self, and stress exposure.[8] Content experts disagree on how the use of empathy affects the development of CF.[49–53] The phenomenon was initially studied in nurses and psychotherapists and is most widely researched in the profession of nursing.[2] The understanding of CF continues to evolve, and there is an increasing call for an updated conceptual model.[2,4,51,54,55] One common conceptualization of CF is the combined effects of burnout and secondary traumatic stress and contrary to CS.[7]

### Burnout

Professional burnout has 3 key dimensions: overwhelming exhaustion, feelings of cynicism or detachment from the job, and a sense of ineffectiveness.[56] Burnout

---

**Box 1**
**Symptoms of compassion fatigue**

- Physical
  - Fatigue
  - Headaches
  - Insomnia

- Behavioral
  - Increased alcohol consumption
  - Absenteeism
  - Impaired clinical decision-making

- Psychological
  - Irritability
  - Relational distancing
  - Emotional exhaustion
  - Negative self-image
  - Depression
  - Anxiety
  - Avoidance
  - Intrusive thoughts
  - Inappropriate reactions
  - Forgetfulness
  - Feeling frustrated, angry, hopeless, disconnected, overwhelmed

- Spiritual
  - Decreased introspection
  - Less discernment

*Data from* Refs.[2–4,7,9]

---

occurs after a person's demands and responsibilities outweigh nourishing and stimulating challenges.[57] The phenomenon may be cyclical in nature, as physical and mental exhaustion can be both symptoms and contributing factors.[57] The mental health ramifications can be severe, as clinical depression symptoms are highly correlated with burnout.[58] The occurrence of burnout is influenced by personal characteristics, attitudes, and beliefs, as well as organizational processes, structures, and values.[49,56,58] The development of burnout occurs over time and can improve with minor changes in work environments, responsibilities, and time demands.[59]

### Secondary traumatic stress

The concept of secondary traumatic stress was introduced in 1995 as a causative factor of CF, specifically in health care providers.[16] Secondary traumatic stress denotes negative emotions driven by exposure to work-related trauma.[7] Empathy and exposure to others' traumatic experiences are central to developing secondary traumatic stress,[50] both of which are common within health care professions. With secondary traumatic stress, a person in a helping role develops stress reactions that lead to decreased psychological functioning.[48] It is an acute phenomenon that can have prolonged effects, with symptoms occurring after just one event that can negatively affect both physical and mental health.[7,48,59]

### Compassion satisfaction

CF may be offset by CS, which refers to the gratification from being able to do work competently.[7] It can include positive feelings about coworkers and one's ability to contribute to the work environment.[7] CS is characterized by feeling invigorated, proficient, and successful in the work being done. Workers feel that they are making a difference and are motivated to continue providing compassionate care because of the positive reinforcement they receive from their colleagues and patients.[7,51]

### Research with Advanced Practice Registered Nurses

Although it is widely acknowledged that health care workers are at high risk for developing CF, there is an evident gap in the literature regarding how APRNs specifically experience and can address this phenomenon. There is noticeably more published research related to CF in physicians, PAs, and nurses, and it is unclear how much of these data apply to APRNs; although APRNs share some professional responsibilities, care models, and practice settings with these occupations, they hold a unique role. One of the most significant predictors of APRN job satisfaction is autonomy,[14] an aspect that differentiates their occupation from nurses or PAs. An integrative literature review about CF in health care providers found that APRNs are not well represented in published CF research.[4] A recent meta-narrative review of CF within the health care literature only used the professions of nurses, physicians, and counselors in their search of electronic databases.[2] Similarly, a systematic review of acute care settings only mentioned physicians and nurses when reporting the results of a literature search regarding CF, burnout, and secondary traumatic stress.[60]

Research related to CF conducted in the last decade includes APRNs; however, many of the studies categorized them with nurses[61,62] or PAs[47] or had samples with less than 3% APRNs when studying health careproviders.[9,11,63,64] The investigators of a recent literature review report that published research with APRNs and/or PAs is limited, usually has small sample sizes, does not report data on the location or duration of the participants' practices, mostly has cross-sectional and descriptive designs, and lacks a basis in conceptual frameworks.[47] This leaves much to be desired regarding the quality of research that includes APRNs.

The available research indicates that burnout is more prevalent in APRNs than in PAs[46] or physicians.[9] APRNs have high work stress in general[13,64] and the reported prevalence of burnout among APRNs include 19.8%,[65] 26.7%,[63] 38%,[64] and "moderate."[66] Edwards and colleagues[67] conducted a cross-sectional analysis of survey data collected over 21 months from more than 10,000 APRNs, PAs, physicians, and staff working in primary care practices. The investigators found that 20.4% of study participants reported experiencing symptoms of burnout, with clinical staff having higher odds of burnout than nonclinical staff.[67] However, it is unclear how these findings can be interpreted for APRNs because the researchers did not differentiate APRNs from PAs when reporting or analyzing the data.[67]

The literature regarding APRNs focuses on what they provide for the health care profession, patients, and physicians, but there is less research addressing their role satisfaction.[14] The available research indicates that APRN job satisfaction is variable and related to specific features of their work. A survey of nearly 13,000 American APRNs reported high satisfaction associated with their level of autonomy, time spent in patient care, sense of value in what they do, and respect from colleagues.[68] In addition to autonomy and professional collaboration, other research with APRNs also reported satisfaction with benefits, community interaction, time and ability to deliver patient care, and finding challenge in the work performed.[14,69-71] Survey data from 196 APRNs working in dermatology indicate that they are highly satisfied with their quality of training, work/life balance, income, and choice of career, specialty, setting, and geographiclocation.[72] APRNs working in other specialties, settings, and locations may be less content with their roles, as other research has reported minimal overall job satisfaction.[69-71] For example, in a study with 181 Midwestern American APRNs, 39.4% were unsure about staying in their current position or intended to leave because of their high stress levels and low job satisfaction.[13] A recent literature review found that studies with APRNs have disproportionately concentrated on job satisfaction versus burnout and turnover.[47] Consequently, there is a paucity of available research related to the development and consequences of CF in APRNs.

### Contributing Factors for Advanced Practice Registered Nurses Developing Compassion Fatigue

The common conceptual model of CF as the combined negative effects of burnout and secondary traumatic stress has noted limitations; for example, it does not include a description of how CF or CS develops or is related to the professional environment.[51] Another proposed model of CF suggests that the process of developing CF or CS corresponds to the balance of resources, utilization of empathy, and appraisal of stress.[51] This model identifies the antecedents to be related to the work environment, client, caregiver, and clinical features.[51] These aspects are related to a professional quality of life framework composed of 3 domains: the work, the client, and person environments[7]; each of these conditions can influence workers' levels of CF and CS.

### The work environment

The work environment of APRNs, which includes their required tasks and employment organization's features, can create situational stressors that promote the development of CF. In the 1970s, APRNs expressed dissatisfaction related to the shortage of opportunities for advancement and lack of administrative support.[73] More recent research indicates that APRNs continue to experience difficulties related to interprofessional, organizational, and policy aspects, all of which can contribute to CF. APRNs from 19 countries reported a perceived lack of respect from physicians and supervisors.[74] APRNs in the United States report dissatisfaction with collegial relationships, administrative support, and organizational leadership.[13,64,69,70] APRN job satisfaction lessens with inadequate resources to treat patients, chaotic work environments, and low levels of perceived work control.[14,64,73,75] Aspects of using an electronic health record can also increase APRN burnout, as it can cause daily frustration and require time spent at home documenting due to insufficient allotted documentation time during the workday.[64,65] APRNs report difficulty with maintaining work-life balance and a desire to be given more time for research and professional service activities.[14,71] Furthermore, APRN faculty report that their positions entail many expectations and responsibilities that do not align with what is rewarded in their academic environment.[76]

It is reasonable to assume that APRNs who work in similar practice settings and in analogous roles to other professionals may share commonalities in the way they develop CF. For example, it is within the scope of psychiatric mental health APRNs to provide psychotherapy. Research with psychotherapists suggests that high caseload volume, engaging only in long-term or individual therapy, and practicing in institutional work settings can negatively affect professional quality of life.[52] A recent systematic review and meta-analysis examining burnout in mental health professionals, including psychotherapists but not specially APRNs, found that workload and professional relationships are key causative factors, whereas role clarity, professional autonomy, perceived fair treatment, and regular supervision are protective factors.[41]

A proposed updated model of CF developed after an integrative literature review suggests that nurses' risk factors for CF include inadequate resources and insufficient positive feedback,[51] and this may also be the case for APRNs. The former National President of the Australian College of Nurse Practitioners stated that it would be naïve to believe that APRNs are not similarly affected by burnout as nurses.[77] Because of the current dearth of published research with APRNs, it is ill-understood if symptoms of CF experienced as a nurse can carry over to subsequent work as an APRN.

### The client environment

Working with patients and their families could be a strong risk factor for APRNs to develop CF. Recent concept analyses of CF within the nursing profession report that contributing factors include intense and prolonged contact with patients, exposure to others' suffering, and the therapeutic use of self when providing care[8,78]; these aspects are also components of APRN practice in various specialties. The lack of research addressing how APRNs' patients can affect levels of CF or CS is notable, as secondary traumatic stress has been documented in other health careprofessionals,[16,48,50,79] so it is reasonable to assume that caring for patients also affects APRNs.

Providing patient care may also be protective against developing CF. National survey data from nearly 13,000 American APRNs reported that the time spent providing patient care was a central aspect of their satisfaction with their jobs.[68] Similarly, a study using a grounded theory approach with 15 American APRNs working in a variety of settings found that building therapeutic relationships with patients was a determining factor in their job satisfaction.[73] Further, data from 120 family APRNs working in Kansas and Missouri indicated that their job satisfaction was highly associated with their time directly caring for patients and their ability to provide quality care.[71]

### The person environment

The third domain of professional quality of life is the person, referring to the APRN's actions and personal characteristics. It is not clear how the amount of professional experience is associated with CF levels, as published research suggests positive,[63,75] neutral,[70] and negative[2,69,71] correlations for health care professionals. One suggested model proposes that a nurse's individual response to personal distress can influence risk of developing CF,[51] and the same may be true of nurses working in an advanced practice role. Burnout is associated with personality traits such as neuroticism and extroversion, which may be more influential in the development of burnout than work-related variables.[58] Meta-analysis data indicate that gender, marital status, and children are sociodemographic variables that significantly correlate with burnout levels in nurses, with single or divorced men with no children having the highest risk.[80] These personal factors may be moderated by age and professional experience, seniority, and satisfaction.[80] Analogous research needs to be conducted with APRNs to examine if there are demographic factors that increase the risk of developing CF.

APRNs' actions can have positive effects on their professional quality of life as well. Published research with more than 200 APRNs and other nursing staff indicates that engagement in health promotional activities is inversely related to CF and burnout and positively correlated with CS.[62] Other actions outside of work may also be significant; research with inpatient providers, including APRNs, suggests that health care professionals who have more personal stressors have higher levels of clinical stress and CF.[79] Therefore, managing personal stress may be helpful in mitigating work-related stress. As with the other domains of professional quality of life, more research is needed that explores how the personal characteristics and behaviors of APRNs influence their levels of CF and CS.

### Potential Interventions

CF in health care providers has the potential to be detrimental for the professional and his or her patients. Investing time and financial resources into targeted interventions could not only improve the professional quality of life of APRNs but also decrease costs related to staff turnover and compromised quality of patient care. A recent systematic review and meta-analysis found 2617 articles related to preventing and reducing physician burnout[81]; unfortunately, there has not been equitable emphasis placed on APRNs. Evidence-based interventions to address CF and its components fall into 2 principal categories: individual and organizational (**Box 2**). The available literature suggests that on an individual basis, APRNs should reflect on their own tolerance for stress[82] and engage in self-care, health promotion, resiliency, and mindfulness activities.[4,62,83,84] Interventions that target health care workers' professional environments at a systems level can also promote and maintain their physical and mental wellbeing.[85] The available research suggests that potential strategies include improving APRNs' job satisfaction[12,69,71,73,74,86–88] and providing educational programs to promote CF awareness, self-care, resilience, mindfulness, relaxation, and coping with emotional distress and difficult patients.[60,63,79,87–92] Incorporating flexibility, sustained employee involvement, and ongoing evaluation regarding barriers and facilitators to participation can promote the success of health care organization interventions.[85]

## Further Exploration

APRNs are a growing and vital part of the health care workforce, and supporting their professional quality of life can promote the value and efficiency of patient care. Although the nursing and physician literature may hold potential insights into the phenomenon of CF within advanced nursing practice, it is essential to conduct more APRN-specific research. Future research endeavors should concentrate on the 2 central reasons for the limited knowledge related to CF in APRNs: the lack of conceptual clarity of CF and the shortage of published research about CF in APRNs particularly.

---

**Box 2**
**Interventions for compassion fatigue in advanced practice registered nurses**

- Individual
  - Meditation
  - Exercise
  - Yoga
  - Counseling
  - Engaging in mindfulness
  - Constructing a support network
- Organizational
  - Increasing nurse practitioner job satisfaction
    - Promoting empowerment
    - Respecting professional values
    - Decreasing weekly work hours
    - Modifying work and break schedules
    - Ensuring adequate appointment times
    - Increasing monetary compensation
    - Mentorship programs
    - Ensuring adequate administrative resources
    - Increasing opportunities for research
    - Widening scope of practice
  - Offering educational programs related to compassion fatigue, emotional distress, dealing with difficult patients, communication skills, resiliency, relaxation, mindfulness

*Data from* Refs.[4,11,12,60,62,69,71,73,74,79,83–88,92]

Fortunately, these 2 aims may both be addressed in the same studies. Given the variety of health care professions and work settings, it is unlikely that there is a single, universally applicable conceptual model of CF.[2] Therefore, continued research to improve the conceptual clarity of CF as it applies to APRNs would aid in better understanding the causes, protective factors, measurement, and effective interventions. Further, conceptual analysis efforts should be specialty specific, as variance in work settings, professional duties, and patient populations may affect how CF is both developed and experienced. As our understanding of how professional burnout and secondary traumatic stress develop is still evolving, additional studies regarding its association with personality traits and work-related factors for APRNs is critical. In addition, longitudinal studies would add in understanding how CF occurs and can change over time.

Implementing and studying interventions for CF should be performed at individual and organizational levels for APRNs of various specialties. Health care organizations should enact targeted interventions to improve the professional quality of life of APRNs and study the effects on providers and patients. Furthermore, local APRN groups can offer opportunities for discussion and education regarding the symptoms, contributing factors, and potential solutions related to CF. These research and intervention efforts are essential to promote a physically, emotionally, and mentally healthy APRN workforce that provides high-quality, efficient health care for patients across the lifespan.

## REFERENCES

1. American Association of Nurse Practitioners. NP facts. 2018. Available at:https://www.aanp.org/images/documents/about-nps/npfacts.pdf. . Accessed December 23, 2018.
2. Sinclair S, Raffin-Bouchal S, Venturato L, et al. Compassion fatigue: a meta-narrative review of the healthcare literature. Int J Nurs Stud 2017;69:9–24.
3. Panagioti M, Geraghty K, Johnson J, et al. Association between physician burnout and patient safety, professionalism, and patient satisfaction: a systematic review and meta-analysis. JAMA Intern Med 2018. https://doi.org/10.1001/jamainternmed.2018.3713.
4. Sorenson C, Bolick B, Wright K, et al. Understanding compassion fatigue in healthcare providers: a review of current literature. J NursScholarsh 2016;48(5):456–65.
5. Bodenheimer T, Sinsky C. From triple to quadruple aim: care of the patient requires care of the provider. Ann Fam Med 2014;12(6):573–6.
6. Institute for Healthcare Improvement. The IHI triple aim. 2018. Available at:http://www.ihi.org/Engage/Initiatives/TripleAim/Pages/default.aspx. . Accessed October 10, 2018.
7. Stamm BH. The concise ProQOL manual. 2nd edition. Pocatello (Idaho): ProQOL.org; 2010.
8. Coetzee SK, Klopper HC. Compassion fatigue within nursing practice: a concept analysis. NursHealthSci 2010;12:235–43.
9. Profit J, Sharek PJ, Amspoker AB, et al. Burnout in the NICU setting and its relation to safety culture. BMJOpenQual 2014;23(10):806–13.
10. Jarrad R, Hammad S, Shawashi T, et al. Compassion fatigue and substance use among nurses. Ann Gen Psychiatry 2018;17(13):1–8.
11. Tawfik DS, Sexton JB, Kan P, et al. Burnout in the neonatal intensive care unit and its relation to healthcare-associated infections. J Perinatol 2017;37(3):315–20.

12. Poghosyan L, Liu J, Shang J, et al. Practice environments and job satisfaction and turnover intentions of nurse practitioners: implications for primary care workforce capacity. HealthCareManage Rev 2017;42(2):162–71.
13. Brom HM, Melnyk BM, Szalacha LA, et al. Nurse practitioners' role perception, stress, satisfaction, and intent to stay at a Midwestern academic medical center. J Am AssocNursePract 2016;28:269–76.
14. De Milt DG, Fitzpatrick JJ, McNulty R. Nurse practitioners' job satisfaction and intent to leave current positions, the nursing profession, and the nurse practitioner role as a direct care provider. J Am AcadNursePract 2011;23: 42–50.
15. Joinson C. Coping with compassion fatigue. Nursing 1992;22(4):116–21.
16. Figley CR. Compassion fatigue: coping with secondary traumatic stress disorder in those who treat the traumatized. New York: Brummer/Mazel; 1995.
17. Bozgeyikli H. Psychological needs as the working-life quality predictor of special education teachers. Uni J Educ Res 2018;6(2):289–95.
18. Sestili C, Scalingi S, Cianfanelli S, et al. Reliability and use of Copenhagen Burnout Inventory in Italian sample of university professors. Int J Environ Res PublicHealth 2018;15(8):1708.
19. Fye HJ, Gnilka PB, McLaulin SE. Perfectionism and school counselors: differences in stress, coping, and burnout. J CounselDev 2018;96:349–60.
20. Talavera-Velasco B, Luceño-Moreno L, Martín-García J, et al. Psychosocial risk factors, burnout and hardy personality as variables associated with mental health in police officers. Front Psychol 2018;9:1–9.
21. Finzi-Dottan R, Kormosh MB. The spillover of compassion fatigue into marital quality: a mediation model. Traumatol 2018;24(2):113–22.
22. Noullet CJ, Lating JM, Kirkhart MW, et al. Effect of pastoral crisis intervention training on resilience and compassion fatigue in clergy: a pilot study. Spiritual Clin Prac 2018;5(1):1–7.
23. Yang F, Li XD, Song ZY, et al. Job burnout of construction project managers: considering the role of organizational justice. J ConstrEngManag 2018;144(11).
24. Truchot D, Andela M. Burnout and hopelessness among farmers: the Farmers Stressors Inventory. SocPsychiatryPsychiatrEpidemiol 2018;53(8):859–67.
25. Delgadillo J, Saxon D, Barkharm M. Association between therapist' occupational burnout and their patients' depression and anxiety treatment outcomes. Depress Anxiety 2018;35(9):844–50.
26. Polachek AJ, Wallace JE. The paradox of compassionate work: a mixed-methods study of satisfying and fatiguing experiences of animal health care providers. Anxiety Stress Coping 2018;31(2):228–43.
27. Rohlf VI. Interventions for occupational stress and compassion fatigue in animal care professionals: a systematic review. Traumatol 2018;24(3):186–92.
28. Garinger LM. The effect of perceived stress and specialization on the relationship between perfectionism and burnout in collegiate athletes. Anxiety Stress Coping 2018. https://doi.org/10.1080/10615806.2018.1521514.
29. WolkowAP, BargerL, O'BrienC, et al.The impact of sleep disturbances and mental health outcomes on burnout in firefighters and the mediating role of sleep during overnight work: a cross-sectional study. 24th Congress of the European Sleep Research Society.Basel, Switzerland, September 25, 2018.
30. Wrzesinska M, Binder K, Tabala K, et al. Burnout and quality of life among massage therapists with visual impairment. J OccupRehabil 2018. https://doi.org/10.1007/s10926-018-9793-7.

31. Ghesquiere A, Plichta SB, McAfee C, et al. Professional quality of life of adult protective service workers. J Elder AbuseNegl 2018;30(1):1–19.

32. Miller JJ, Donohue-Dioh J, Niu C, et al. Exploring the self-care practices of child welfare workers: a research brief. Child YouthServ Rev 2018;84:137–42.

33. Mason HD. The relationship between existential attitudes and professional quality of life among nursing students. J PsycholAfr 2018;28(3):233–6.

34. Tucker T, Bouvette M, Daly S, et al. Finding the sweet spot: developing, implementing and evaluating a burn out and compassion fatigue intervention for third year medical trainees. EvalProgramPlann 2017;65:106–12.

35. Nevins CM, Sherman J, Canchola K, et al. Influencing exercise and hydration self-care practices of baccalaureate nursing students. J Holist Nurs 2018. https://doi.org/10.1177/089801011187922781.

36. Higuchi Y, Inagaki M, Koyama T, et al. A cross-sectional study of psychological distress, burnout, and the associated risk factors in hospital pharmacists in Japan. BMC Public Health 2016;16(1):1–8.

37. Aisling M, Aisling D, Curran D. An assessment of psychological need in emergency medical staff in the Northern Health and Social Care trust area. Ulster Med J 2016;85(2):92–8.

38. Williams B, Lau R, Thornton E, et al. The relationship between empathy and burnout - lessions for paramedics: a scoping review. Psychol Res BehavManag 2017;10:329–37.

39. Singh NN, Lancioni GE, Medvedev ON, et al. Comparative effectiveness of caregiver training in mindfulness-based positive behavior support (MBPBS) and positive behavior support (PBS) in a randomized controlled trial. Mindfulness 2018. https://doi.org/10.1007/s12671-018-0895-2.

40. Kiley KA, Sehgal AR, Neth S, et al. The effectiveness of guided imagery in treating compassion fatigue and anxiety of mental health workers. SocWork Res 2018; 42(1):33–43.

41. O'Connor K, Neff DM, Pitman S. Burnout in mental health professionals: a systematic review and meta-analysis of prevalence and determinants. EurPsychiatry 2018;53:74–99.

42. Silver J, Caleshu C, Casson-Parkin S, et al. Mindfulness among genetic counselors is associated with increased empathy and work engagement and decreased burnout and compassion fatigue. J Genet Couns 2018;27: 1175–86.

43. Reis H, Vale C, Camacho C, et al. Burnout among occupational therapists in Portugal: a study of specific factors. OccupTherHealthCare 2018. https://doi.org/10.1080/07380577.2018.1497244.

44. Aquino E, Lee Y, Spawn N, et al. The impact of burnout on doctorate nursing faculty's intent to leave their academic position: a descriptive survey research design. NurseEducToday 2018;69(35–40).

45. Zhang Y, Zhang C, Han X, et al. Determinants of compassion satisfaction, compassion fatigue and burn out in nursing: a correlative meta-analysis. Medicine 2018;97(26):e11086.

46. Coplan B, McCall TC, Smith N, et al. Burnout, job satisfaction, and stress levels of PAs. JAAPA 2018;31(9):42–6.

47. Hoff T, Carabetta S, Collinson GE. Satisfaction, burnout, and turnover among nurse practitioners and physician assistants: a review of the empirical literature. Med Care Res Rev 2017. https://doi.org/10.1177/1077558717730157.

48. Thomas RB, Wilson JP. Issues and controversies in the understanding and diagnosis of compassion fatigue, vicarious traumatization, and secondary traumatic stress disorder. Int J EmergMentHealth 2004;6(2):81–92.
49. Sabo B. Reflecting on the concept of compassion fatigue. Online J IssuesNurs 2011;16(1):1.
50. Beck CT. Secondary traumatic stress in nurses: a systematic review. Arch PsychiatrNurs 2011;25(1):1–10.
51. Coetzee SK, Laschinger HKS. Toward a comprehensive, theoretical model of compassion fatigue: an integrative literature review. NursHealthSci 2018; 20(1):4–15.
52. Laverdiere O, Kealy D, Ogrodniczuk JS. Psychotherapists' professional quality of life. Traumatol 2018. https://doi.org/10.1037/trm0000177.
53. Hansen EM, Eklund JH, Hallen A, et al. Does feeling empathy lead to compassion fatigue or compassion satisfaction?The role of time perspective. J Psychol 2018. https://doi.org/10.1080/00223980.2018.1495170.
54. Gerard N. Rethinking compassion fatigue. J HealthOrganManag 2017;31(3): 363–8.
55. Sorenson C, Bolick B, Wright K, et al. An evolutionary concept analysis of compassion fatigue. J NursScholarsh 2017;49(5):557–63.
56. Maslach C, Schaufeli WB, Leiter MP. Job burnout. Annu Rev Psychol 2001;52: 397–422.
57. Ekstedt M, Fagerberg I. Lived experiences of the time preceding burnout. J AdvNurs 2005;49(1):59–67.
58. Bianchi R, Mayor E, Schonfeld IS, et al. Burnout and depressive symptoms are not primarily linked to perceived organizational problems. PsycholHealth Med 2018;23(9):1094–105.
59. Branson DC. Vicarious trauma, themes in research, and terminology: a review of the literature. Traumatol 2018. https://doi.org/10.1037/trm0000161.
60. van Mol MMC, Kompanje EJO, Benoit DD, et al. The prevalence of compassion fatigue and burnout among healthcare professionals in intensive care units: a systematic review. PLoS One 2015;10(8):e0136955.
61. Branch C, Klinkenberg D. Compassion fatigue among pediatric healthcare providers. MCN Am J Matern Child Nurs 2015;40(3):160–6.
62. Neville K, Cole DA. The relationships among health promotion behaviors, compassion fatigue, burnout, and compassion satisfaction in nurses practicing in a community medical center. J NursAdm 2013;43(6):348–54.
63. Tawfik DS, Phibbs CS, Sexton JB, et al. Factors associated with provider burnout in the NICU. J Pediatr 2017;139(5):1–9.
64. Linzer M, Poplau S, Babbott S, et al. Worklife and wellness in academic general internal medicine: results from a national survey. J Gen Intern Med 2016;31(9): 1004–10.
65. Harris DA, Haskell J, Cooper E, et al. Estimating the association between burnout and electronic health record related stress among advanced practice registered nurses. ApplNurs Res 2018;43:36–41.
66. Geelan-Hansen K, Anne S, Benninger MS. Burnout in otolaryngology-head and neck surgery: a single academic center experience. OtolaryngolHeadNeckSurg 2018;159(2):254–7.
67. Edwards ST, Marino M, Balasubramanian BA, et al. Burnout among physicians, advanced practice clinicians and staff in smaller primary care practices. J Gen Intern Med 2018;33(12):2138–46.

68. Chattopadhyay A, Zangaro GA, White KM. Practice patterns and characteristics of nurse practitioners in the United States: results from the 2012 national sample survey of nurse practitioners. J NursePract 2015;11(2):170–7.
69. Faris JA, Douglas MK, Maples DC, et al. Job satisfaction of advanced practice nurses in the Veterans Health Administration. J Am AcadNursePract 2010; 22(1):35–44.
70. Pasaron R. Nurse practitioner job satisfaction: looking for successful outcomes. J ClinNurs 2013;22:2593–604.
71. Ryan ME, Ebbert DW. Nurse practitioner satisfaction: identifying perceived beliefs and barriers. J NursePract 2013;9(7):428–34.
72. Cheng CE, Kimball AB, VanCott A. A survey of dermatology nurse practitioners: work setting, training, and job satisfaction. J DermatolNursesAssoc 2010;2(1): 19–23.
73. Shea ML. Determined persistence: achieving and sustaining job satisfaction among nurse practitioners. J Am AssocNursePract 2015;27(1):31–8.
74. Steinke MK, Rogers M, Lehwaldt D, et al. An examination of advanced practice nurses' job satisfaction internationally. IntNurs Rev 2018;65(2):162–72.
75. Whitebird RR, Solberg LI, Crain AL, et al. Clinician burnout and satisfaction with resources in caring for complex patients. Gen HospPsychiatry 2017;44:91–5.
76. Fontenot HB, Hawkins JW, Weiss JA. Cognitive dissonance experienced by nurse practitioner faculty. J Am AcadNursePract 2012;24:506–13.
77. Raftery C. Nurse practitioners: Do we care? J NursePract 2015;11(6):653.
78. Jenkins B, Warren N. Concept analysis: compassion fatigue and effects upon critical care nurses. CritCareNurs Q 2012;35(4):388–95.
79. Meadors J, Lamson A. Compassion fatigue and secondary traumatization: provider self care on intensive care units for children. J PediatrHealthCare 2008; 22(1):24–34.
80. Cañadas-De la Fuente GA, Ortega E, Ramirez-Baena L, et al. Gender, marital status, and children as risk factors for burnout in nurses: a meta-analytic study. Int J Environ Res PublicHealth 2018;15(10):1–13.
81. West CPD, Liselotte N, Erwin PJ, et al. Interventions to prevent and reduce physician burnout: a systematic review and meta-analysis. Lancet 2016;388:2272–81.
82. Edmunds MW. Growth in NP role satisfaction may have limits. J NursePract 2014; 10(1):A9–10.
83. Harolds JA. Quality and safety in healthcare, Part XLVII: resilience and burnout. ClinNucl Med 2018. https://doi.org/10.1097/RLU.0000000000002303.
84. Lomas T, Medina JC, Ivtzan I, et al. A systematic review of the impact of mindfulness on the well-being of healthcare professionals. J ClinPsychol 2017;74: 319–55.
85. Brand SL, Coon JT, Fleming LE, et al. Whole-system approaches to improving the health and wellbeing of healthcare workers: a systematic review. PLoS One 2017; 12(12):e1088418.
86. Stewart JG, McNulty R, Griffin MTQ, et al. Psychological empowerment and structural empowerment among nurse practitioners. J Am AcadNursePract 2010;22:27–34.
87. Ruotsalainen JH, Verbeek JH, Marine A, et al. Preventing occupational stress in healthcare settings. CochraneDatabaseSyst Rev 2015;(4):CD002892.
88. Hall LH, Johnson J, Heyhoe J, et al. Strategies to improve general practitioner well-being: findings from a focus group study. FamPract 2018;35(4):511–6.

89. Edgoose JY, Regner CJ, Zakletskaia LI. BREATHE OUT: a randomized controlled trial of a structured intervention to improve clinician satisfaction with "difficult" visits. J Am BoardFam Med 2015;28(1):13–20.
90. Klein CJ, Riggenbach-Hays JJ, Sollenberger LM, et al. Quality of life and compassion satisfaction in clinicians: a pilot intervention study for reducing compassion fatigue. Am J HospPalliatCare 2018;35(6):882–8.
91. Fortney L, Luchterhand C, Zakletskaia L, et al. Abbreviated mindfulness intervention for job satisfaction, quality of life, and compassion in primary care clinicians: a pilot study. Ann Fam Med 2013;11(5):412–20.
92. Praissman S. Mindfulness-based stress reduction: a literature review and clinician's guide. J Am AcadNursePract 2008;20:212–6.

# *Moving?*

## *Make sure your subscription moves with you!*

To notify us of your new address, find your **Clinics Account Number** (located on your mailing label above your name), and contact customer service at:

**Email: journalscustomerservice-usa@elsevier.com**

**800-654-2452** (subscribers in the U.S. & Canada)
**314-447-8871** (subscribers outside of the U.S. & Canada)

**Fax number: 314-447-8029**

**Elsevier Health Sciences Division**
**Subscription Customer Service**
**3251 Riverport Lane**
**Maryland Heights, MO 63043**

*To ensure uninterrupted delivery of your subscription, please notify us at least 4 weeks in advance of move.